Contraption of the Crossroads

George O. Obikoya

Table of Contents

Executive Summary   3

Introduction   6

Of education and health   10

What has the environment to do with health?   37

Who needs drugs companies?   58

What does health matter?   80

A Mystic health voyage   104

Conclusions   125

Executive Summary

That health spending is increasing faster than incomes in most developed

countries is no longer news. Concerns regarding how they fund health services
with the health budget of the U.S for example projected to double in a decade, to
$4.1 trillion, half paid by the federal government, however also continue to grow.
This is more so, as many of these countries increasingly question the value
derived from their soaring health bills. Is something missing somewhere is why
we have what many would consider a healthcare crisis even in developed
countries? Should we not zealously seek answers to this and other questions
crucial to fixing our health systems to minimize if not avert the potential adverse

consequences for not just us, but also our entire economy, more so in an increasingly competitive global marketplace?

Yet, how much of a country's gross domestic product (GDP), essentially a measure of it wealth, it could afford to spend on healthcare is an important consideration. With health care spending globally is in general increasing faster than overall economic growth, many countries spending more of their wealth on healthcare, it is also pertinent to query the sustainability of ever increasing health spending. The U.S for example spent 8.8% of its GDP on health in 1980, and by 2003, 15.2%, a nearly 7 percentage-point increase in the health share of GDP. In fact, its 2003 health spending per capita was about 90% more than many other developed countries. Should the U.S and indeed, other countries therefore, not be exploring ways to deliver accessible and qualitative healthcare delivery more efficiently and cost-effectively? What policy initiatives would such goals warrant and what are their potential ramifications for other sectors of the economy?

Furthermore, that we should couple practical measures with vision in solving the myriads of problems health systems face worldwide is not in question. Indeed, the former constitutes the general framework apposite to ensuring that the latter materializes. This e-book aims to achieve this objective in an effort to highlight the significant issues that contemporary health systems face relative to the potential for addressing them effectively, to preempt change to which they are subject, compounding the chaos that now tends to propel them along a moribund path. We would therefore in this e-book, embark on an exploration of the underpinnings of qualitative health services provision in an increasingly complex, and competitive milieu, internal and external to the processes whose eventual results could be portentous for all healthcare stakeholders, and for the economy, perhaps even dramatically.

Introduction

It is not always that we find appropriate expressions for the rationale behind our action, which nonetheless we hold with such conviction that nothing would sway us away from it. There are drivers in us that we have little control over, in a sense, but which, ultimately we do, in another. In this regard, we could be wary of the price of freedom, if any, of the randomness of events in our brains impelling us to sacrifice some individuals for the 'good' of many more, or indeed, to eat grass. The point about common sense being antithetical to freedom or otherwise raises concerns over its validity regardless of the randomness or orderliness of its source in the particular decision, and subsequent action in question. Yet these drivers, to the extent that they underlie those decisions are at once deterministic, yet liberating assuring the freedom that they seem on the surface to constrain.

W e need confront and accept the potential that we have to choose between various options with the fundamental tendency of motion to move us in a potentially different direction, within a framework, in fact, of three mutually dependent directions, namely forward, or backward motion, or actually wobbling on the spot, once so acquiesced. The concept of the wobble itself is significant for the dependence on one another of the three options, with the kinesis inherent in us, incompatible with anything else, which itself determines the eventuality of dissipation, on the spot on the one hand, or a backward motion, which the loss of dissipation could also engender in any motion. Thus, the backward motion could originate from the wobble, as it could from a deceleration of the forward motion, transition the wobble, or skip it, into a moribund path.

H ere again, we see the potential of each option to influence the other, and for a coalescence of options on the one hand, and how we could, by the choices we make, influence these processes, on the other. Our exploration of the underpinnings of healthcare delivery in this e-book would thus, reveal the frameworks within which the specific actions that we need to take to improve our health services, and indeed, address the multiplicity of issues confronting them, successfully hinge. We would see in our discussions the interplay of the two in not just the current problems our health services struggle with, but in the solutions to them, as our efforts at teasing out the underlying forces that we should muster in improving the services enable us appreciate fuller, their significance for the initiatives to achieve our goals. It would be clear to us as we proceed that we should not necessarily be short on practicalities having recognized the underlying driving vision for moving our health service forward, but that rather, it is this vision coupled with the initiatives it inspires that would ensure the realization of its elements.

Considering that these revelations would constitute the rudiments of the

forces that would spur us into action, our exploratory tendencies would in effect bear fruit literally of the sort that we crave in the first place to embark on it. That the issues health systems face are generic and specific, each particular health jurisdiction therefore going to have to determine theirs, but also approach the solutions to them from the perspective of the generic, would be self-evident. Again, our exploration would reveal the significance of this perspective, as indeed, perhaps, of a critical missing link in our current approaches, which have evidently not met the expectations of the generality in many health jurisdictions. It is this potential for coupling vision with the outcomes of our ongoing analyses of our health systems, which would not only reveal the most appropriate solutions, but also inspire their implementations in full.

I t therefore seems reasonable to adopt the premise of the need for such an

exploration being the motive for us to conduct it as we propose in this e-book.
The subject matter illustrative of the operations of this coupling would be
eclectic, and some would contend atypical. This itself, underlines the complexity
of the nature of our discourse, and the need for us in attempting to establish the
coupling prepare to venture outside customary domains, since, as is in fact the
case, the forces that shape healthcare delivery, and would increasingly so do,
would situate within and without the health domain. It is thus, the case that the
link between health and economy, in a general sense immediately obvious to
many, being just as important to be so when we deem the need for action
warrants taking measures, in not just the health sector, but in other domains, that
would help in preventing the disruption of the harmony between the two. In the
end, the achievement of our primary objectives, which the exploration that
revealed our vision mandates us to chase, would take precedence over any
measures that would tend to prevent us from so doing, which again, our full
appreciation of the significance of the vision so revealed would spawn.

Of Education and Health

That education plays a key role in our individual and social lives is not in question. The benefits to society of imparting knowledge either formally, in schools, or informally, in sundry settings, many acknowledge and indeed, crave. Few would dispute the need to educate our children to prepare them for the invariably challenging sojourn through life ahead. Not also, many would contend that we all need lifelong education on a variety of issues relevant to our lives, not to mention those we have to deal with as members of a group, community, even country, and as humans. We tend to conceptualize education in general terms, an atavistic relic we cannot ignore, one that nonetheless, limits our perspectives on this vital issue in profound ways, yet surprisingly belies an even deeper contraption of a worldview on its relationship to health that not just undermines the potency of both, but in particular operating in tandem. It is not difficult to see the act and process of imbibing knowledge and skills in both domains separately creating an enabling environment for the achievement of their respective goals. It is a different matter, however, conceptualizing the fundamentals common to both and upon which neither, not predicated, would not eventually wither. There is no gainsaying the eclectic dimensions of education for instance, from musings to discourses, and the transition from the simplistic to the intricate bidirectional in most societies, despite the inherence of the tendency of transition being from the former to the latter as societies become increasingly complex, although as we will argue, desirable, is instructive. Placing the philosophy of education astride developments in multiple domains capable of influencing it therefore, is the persistence of this bidirectional motion, whose significance might not be immediately obvious, other than for example, the moot point about the value of education itself if not perpetual. The point is moot because it is the quality of education, and not its form that really counts, which does not in itself diminish the value of the simplistic mode, but highlights its misdirection viewed naively. Thus, even if oral tradition constitutes the mode of education in less complex societies, it does not necessarily make this educational form, simplistic. Nor does it make that of a more complex society with more structured schooling with teacher and student roles clearly defined, intricate. It is precisely this point we want to establish as the reason for the desirability of the bidirectional transition mentioned earlier. In other words, both the simplistic and intricate forms of education are applicable in every society in the prevailing circumstances. Indeed, it has always been, even if we did not so recognize, and apply this crucial principle, which is why this failure is instructive of a particular mindset that requires overhauling to signify the massive nature of the enterprise before us that we need to ensure meets, perhaps even surpasses the demands of out time. The challenges ahead therefore transcend dichotomous considerations of Lockean tabula rasa, or as Jean-Jacques Rousseau argued in *Emile*, that we are born curious, ready to learn. We are increasingly confronted with dramatic developments in domains out side education, for example, in information and communication technologies, such as the commons-based peer production systems, open-source software development and folksonomy, the magnitude of whose potential influence on how we conceptualize education is yet to become manifest. Yet, this reminds us of a key idea of the Brazilian Paulo Freire (1921-1997) regarding annulling the teacher/student dichotomy, in a democratic infusion into educational practice counter to the outcome of the latter being a key facilitator of the former in general currency. In other words, what would be the significance of such developments as shared vocabulary that users on Del.icio.us, a notable folksonomy website, originate and propagate, for the obscurity inherent in tackling the semantics-from-syntax conundrum a propos 'meaning'? Are such developments reminiscent of the evolution of language on which our evolution, and reality pivot, including the direction of education, and indeed, of all else? Are we seeing a reorientation long overdue of the natural path of democracy, implied as inevitable? What are the potential effects of these developments on health and healthcare delivery? Arguable some would regard them as epiphenomena, of the more fundamental dyadic that education and health constitute, one whose mechanics as earlier noted, we apparently conceptualize so fuzzily that this further encrypts the real issues that we must address, delaying which process as we thus do, with adverse consequences for both education and health that we see all around us. However, let us reflect a little more on these secondary issues, perhaps this would elucidate our ruminations on the more profound ones along the way. Would the flexibility of folksonomies for example, hence their potential for accelerated changes be the defining factor in their evolution into a superior 'taxonomy' as tagging becomes more dependable? Would this be even likelier with for instance the emergence of the Semantic Web, the lure of web pages capable via their machine-readable metadata of describing their contents difficult to resist for even for example, professional groups? What would the effects of the potential compromises between taxonomy and folksonomy, in for example, taxonomy directed folksonomy (TDF) [1], among others be for the widespread diffusion of the latter? Would folksonomies become increasingly a viable information retrieval and organization approach in firms, organizations, and in workplaces in general, and to what extent could they be as they evolve, and would they become so more reliable for employment in tactical and operational situations, and even in strategic management? Given not just being less costly than conventional taxonomies, but the inherent democratic orientation it fosters indispensable to the practices that the operations of the fundamentals mentioned earlier spawn, is this then, as are many others that we would encounter in our discussion, representative of the inevitable process constitutive of the direction the education-health dyadic heads? As we, therefore dig deeper into these issues, it is apposite to leap forward into the realities of our health systems for example, most bogged down by ever-increasing costs that health jurisdictions could clearly ill-afford. To complicate matters, the resulting increased health spending does not seem to make much difference to health indicators in many such jurisdictions. Worse still, we anticipate potential additional increase in health spending due to aging populations in many developed countries for example, or in some developing countries, due to the adverse economic, hence health effects of epidemic diseases, among others. As the latter example shows, the adversity that compromised economic growth and development occasions is unrestricted to certain countries as it is perhaps the degree to which it would manifest that varies. It is thus necessary, and indeed, mandatory for all countries, developing and developed to start to pay more attention to developments within and outside their health sector that could influence healthcare delivery in their countries, including in education. 'Participatory development' in true Freirian tradition, which underscores emancipation via interactive participation is at the core of the paradigmatic shift in healthcare delivery toward the patient being the center of the healthcare delivery universe, so to say. Here, unlike Freire's focus, we are not just talking about the emancipation/ empowerment of the poor, our concern is that of the individual, uncharacterized. This generalized approach to empowerment itself underlines not just the point made earlier regarding the desirability of the simplistic/intricate dichotomy, nullifying which as perceived conventionally, emphasizing instead its validity in stressing content rather than form, buttressing the need for the bidirectional flow of both approaches even in developed countries. In other words, the potential of empowerment in development is realizable to the extent that it is general, not restricted to particular groups, poor or otherwise, which is not the same thing as saying that we could not, and indeed, should not contextualize it. Let us for now restrict our discussions to the higher levels, as this would make 'operationalizing' smoother-going down the road. Thus, if we indeed, considered the individual healthcare consumer the central figure in the entire enterprise, we would expect not just to appreciate the expectations of this consumer regarding healthcare delivery, but actively work toward meeting them. Yet, we could not expect so to do with these expectations haywire, rooted in nothing other than whim. Now, certain basic factors preclude us meeting such idiosyncratic expectations, primarily those economic. Two basic economic principles, that of scarcity, since we could not expect to meet all the needs of everyone all the time, hence and second, the need for rational resource allocation and utilization, mandate us to act prudently, even in meeting the expectations of the individual healthcare consumer. There is no doubt that we could not succeed in so doing without the cooperation of the healthcare consumer. In other words, the healthcare consumer has to be able to collaborate in the first place, but how could we secure this collaboration for example in rational resource utilization if the healthcare consumer lacked the relevant information to assist in taking discerning decisions regarding service utilization? It is therefore clear that one of the first steps that we need to take in acknowledging the significance of the centrality of the healthcare consumer in the healthcare delivery enterprise is to rectify the information asymmetry pervasive in the healthcare industry. However, as we have argued thus far, regarding the desirability of the bi-directionality of the simplistic/intricate approaches to education, it is inherently in the interest of the healthcare consumer expecting the health system to meet his or her needs to create the enabling milieu for meeting those expectations.

The onus therefore is not just on the health system, but also on the healthcare consumer to facilitate, the realization of the expectations of the healthcare consumer, as it is also on the former to ensure the achievements of its stated objectives, including meeting the expectations of the healthcare consumer. These collaborative efforts require interactive processes whose facilitation become urgent in circumstances such as our and this applies essentially to all health systems, where we seem to have stalled in many ways moving healthcare delivery forward. Yet, the motion of healthcare delivery is inherent, even if its direction is conjectural, at least to the extent that we could hardly, from one perspective at least guarantee the nature of the operations of the forces crucial to its motorization in the prevailing circumstances. That it is however, possible that we could is the raison d'etre for the arguments we would advance here, for the crucial interplay of education and health being necessary to comprehend in its appropriate nature and form. To be sure, the motion of healthcare delivery, as of all the processes involved in our very existence could be one of three, forward, backward, or wobbling on the spot. It is arguable if the inherent motion should not be forward, or is it considering the desirability in the main for us to want to live? We could point to examples of communities that have essentially willed themselves in the direction of death, for a variety of reasons, and some would even argue that natural selection encourages this 'backward motion' among those not-so evolutionary fit to survive. It is also arguable whether natural selection accounts for the events in Jonestown, Guyana, or other processes outside the evolutionary mode. The hardly disputable point though is that most of humanity prefers to live. This is evident even in historical terms in the perpetuity of humanity, at least thus far, despite aspects of its constituents being at some point moribund, even extinct. This is not to say that the backward motion could not be sufficiently pervasive among its constituent parts to pose significant threats to the very survival of the entire entity. Indeed, it has come close to such situations even as recently as during the Cuban missile crisis of the early 1960s, the point of whose outcome buttresses this proclivity to survive in the generality than otherwise, one could argue. So then, it is the forward motion that is likely preeminent in the options presented earlier, which is the point about being able to control it, as this makes such control much easier to achieve, or does it? The question is appropriate considering the potential for such control that we seem to continue to fritter, despite our levels of sophistication intellectually, relative to the past, in the sheer numbers for examples, of the educated, which encompasses the literate or otherwise. This again stresses, the bi-directionality mentioned earlier, in both its form and context, being the critical issue, rather the dichotomy of one versus the other, as it is evident that neither has met its goals. The conclusion is apt if we concurred with us, not yet being able to control the direction of healthcare delivery, as we ought to, for example, in the forward path. Thus education, whether simplistic, or intricate, has not sufficiently equipped us with the resources to appreciate the things we really ought to do to move our health systems forward. The question then is what we really ought to do to achieve this objective. The answer is what we would consider the ingredient of a novel conceptualization of the education/health dyadic appropriate to the changing milieu in which we deliver healthcare on the one hand and its relationships to the entirety of that in which it operates singly, and in tandem with other systems, on the other. The education of the healthcare consumer therefore, has to be bi-directional, in other words both simplistic and intricate, because we do not have the time to spare having delayed progress of the forward motion, not having done what we should have to move it forward fast enough. This delay is tantamount to the motion wobbling on the spot, which is therefore currently the case, and which worse still, could transition into backward motion, if we did not expedite action on moving it forward. Thus, we want to avoid as much as possible the transience of the wobbly motion, as backward motion would be even harder to transform into forward motion. What then do we mean by the education being bi-directional the most appropriate way to move the motion forward? First, having concurred that the pervasive information asymmetry in the health sector is compromising the ability of the healthcare consumer, who we have placed at the center of our healthcare delivery universe, literally-speaking, to take discerning healthcare decisions crucial to the forward motion of our health systems, we need to rectify it. In so doing, we must acknowledge the disparities in educational levels, and in the abilities of healthcare consumers to acquire and imbibe information in every society. In other words, even in the highly literate societies, there are still individuals with disparities along these dimensions. The need to cater for these different groups of persons is therefore, real, and their requirements, variable. We need therefore, to employ appropriate measures, simplistic and intricate in rectifying information asymmetry, which underscores the point made earlier about the obligation of all healthcare stakeholders, including the healthcare consumer, in this and other issues regarding moving our health systems forward. In this regard, it would be necessary therefore, for the healthcare consumer to be willing to adopt the healthcare information and communication technologies (healthcare ICT), for example, that could help achieve the goal of rectifying information asymmetry at both the simplistic and intricate levels. This might sound contradictory to some, considering these technologies perhaps generally seen as appropriate for the intricate form of education, rather than the simplistic. However, if we agreed that such an assumption reflects a dichotomous approach to education, we would not only see the relevance of these technologies in the so-called simplistic approach, but the significance of the bi-directional perspective that we thus far emphasized. Indeed, many developing countries are bypassing conventionality and adopting these technologies despite a significant lack of technological and other infrastructures, making the applicability of the dichotomy irrelevant even in settings where they would have otherwise. In a similar vein, it is not the case that everyone in the developed countries has access to these technologies. These issues clearly highlight the need for embracing the bi-directionality of simplistic/intricate approaches to education in addressing the information asymmetry issue. The nature, form, and content of the initiatives in particularly health jurisdictions would however, have to depend on local details, formulated within this general framework. Thus, each health jurisdiction would be able to determine the relative importance in particular initiatives of its goals in inculcating health information, news, and knowledge, promoting intellectual independence in acquiring and using such information and knowledge, and in value building or otherwise, in the ethico-moral and political domains, all crucial to the evolution of our health systems. The appropriateness of the initiatives would manifest in the enhanced knowledge of the operations of the health systems, itself reflected in the in the decisions taking regarding their utilization for example, with regards the healthcare consumer, and in optimal resource allocation and utilization, for example, with regards healthcare providers, both predicated on the availability of timely and accurate information. The healthcare consumer for example would be able to recognize the worsening of the wait lists issue his or her not showing up for a scheduled appointment with the doctor , and not canceling the appointment prior, could potentially cause, including in fact, the costs in material and human terms. The healthcare provider/system on the other hand would realize the benefits to improving the wait lists problem making information available on doctors that could assist the healthcare provider in scheduling such appointments in the first place. Both the healthcare consumer that desires accelerated physician consultation, and the healthcare provider /system losing money and goodwill because of long wait lists, would have met their stated objectives. Indeed, the improved balance in information flow between the two would encourage the sort of dialogue and consultation that would, for example enable the healthcare consumer to appreciate the transparency of his or her healthcare jurisdiction in tackling problems in the jurisdiction, for example, in expanding/closing services, and in even outsourcing nonviable services, and in taking other measures. This would be even more so as such dialogue would have made it possible for the healthcare consumer, or his or here representative on the appropriate consultative committee to be part of the decision-making process, a democratic approach to addressing healthcare delivery issues that is inevitable in all health jurisdictions to move them forward. This instillation of political, and of ethico-moral, values should be part of the goals of education mentioned above, and is critical to achieve from an early age in an individual, hence another reason to embrace the bi-directionality of educational approaches to move our health systems forward. In other words, the engagement of the person, no matter how simplistic, from an early age regarding the elements of health, its value, and aspects of healthcare delivery, is sine qua non to that individual appreciating the novel conceptualizations of these issues here discussed in totality. This appreciation on the other hand, if pervasive, and which should be the goal, would be the stimulus for continued positive approaches to health system resource allocation and utilization, the two key underlying economic principles mentioned above, that constitute the essential ingredients of our abilities to meet the likely increasingly sophisticated expectations of our peoples of their health systems.

Thus, the interaction of the knowledge acquired in the simplistic mode with

that acquired in the intricate mode would be an ongoing exercise in every health jurisdiction, the relative weight given either hence would necessarily have a local flavor. Thus, we conceptualize education in ways that would enable us acquire different heuristics perspectives that could help us move our health systems only pragmatically if they did. Without bogging down the discussion with the peculiarities of pragmatism, suffice to emphasize the crucial appropriate operations of the individual/community dyadic in the forward motion that we intend to achieve. In other words, just as we concluded with the simplistic/intricate dyadic, the issue is not dichotomizing which component of this individual/community dyadic is superior to the other, even taking the matter that far. On the other hand, we want to place the interests of each at par, and move the health system forward. This pragmatism, we want to argue works for both, eschewing the classical utilitarian dimensions on the one hand, and the Rawlian, on the other. In other words, the desire of the individual to survive coincides with the interests of the community in so doing, and no initiative that we set forth would have achieved the goal of moving the health system were it bereft of such fundamentals, which would be evident in a lack of consensus on health resource allocation/utilization for example. This again emphasizes the need for education in rectifying the information asymmetry that would make such consensus difficult to arrive at. Our conceptualization of education as a key driver of the motion of healthcare delivery has important dimensions for the health systems as well. In being discerning in the use of health services for example, individuals would be helping to reduce healthcare costs, hence health spending, by both themselves, and by the health system. This is regardless of the health financing model of the particular health jurisdiction, although the tilt of the benefits would vary based on this mode, some would argue, more for the health system, and for the healthcare consumer, in publicly, and privately financed health systems, respectively, for examples, at least on the surface. In other words, the cumulative effects of the rational allocation and use of scarce healthcare resources is not just in the interests of the healthcare consumer, or the health systems, but rather in the interests of both. There is no doubt that that the healthcare consumer in the U.S., for example, would spend, at least in theory, less on health services provision, if more discerning, and in a publicly funded health system as in Canada, the health system would, if individuals use services less. The crucial issue besides adhering strictly to economic principles to ensure the survival of the health system and to move it forward is ensuring the delivery of qualitative services accessible to all. No health system could afford to ignore both issues, as the increase in illness prevalence that would ensure not ensuring such high quality and accessible services, would in turn escalate healthcare costs, and spending. With health spending on the increase perpetually, it would be even more difficult to meet the expectations of the peoples of their health systems, more peoples would become ill and costs would further increase, a vicious cycle no health system could afford. In fact, no country could, considering the overall effects of the health system sliding backward on other aspects of the economy. The goals of our health systems would therefore likely increasingly be dual, what we would call the dual healthcare delivery objectives (DHDO), the delivery of qualitative health services without increasing, health spending, and in fact, decreasing it, essentially. This takes us to another dimension of our conceptualization of the important role of education in health, and healthcare delivery, which is in the achievement of the DHDO. Thus, education also drives the motion of healthcare delivery in helping us achieve the delivery of qualitative health services, efficiently and cost-effectively, an extension of the earlier dimensions discussed. This extension also has simplistic and intricate dimensions, as the achievement of the delivery of such services predicates on the interactive dyadic between the healthcare consumer and the health system operating efficiently and cost-effectively. Thus we could not expect the senior that has diabetes and heart disease to know for example, that he or she does not have to worry about the difficulty getting to the hospital for their appointments to see the specialists if they lacked the knowledge that healthcare

ICT is available that could enable domiciliary consultation and treatment for example. Yet, the senior does not have didactics to acquire such knowledge even if he or she lived in a developed country. It is also important for example, for the healthcare consumer to be part of the electronic health records (EHR) systems burgeoning in a health jurisdiction say, were such systems to achieve their full functional potential. Besides the enormous resources invested in the implementation of such technologies potentially coming to naught, we would not have been able for example to enable the healthcare consumer benefit from the availability at the point of care (POC) of current and accurate information in real time that could prove vital in saving the healthcare consumer's life. This would be the case as in this situation if the healthcare provider did not hookup to the EHR because he or she did not know of or adopt the technologies required for such information provision. Even in not ensuring that he or she receives the most appropriate treatment, we might be prolonging the illness in question in ways that would incur significant costs in human and material terms. In both examples given above, we could be further increasing healthcare costs and spending, by our inactions, or flawed actions, evidence of which abound now, considering the slow pace of the adoption of healthcare ICT for example, by not just the healthcare consumer, but also by the healthcare provider, and indeed, by all healthcare stakeholders. Here again, education plays a key role in increasing the appreciation for example, for these technologies as means by which we could facilitate the achievement of the dual healthcare delivery objectives (DHDO), in which we all have a stake. Most crucially, started at an early age, in the simplistic mode mentioned earlier, and as it evolves into the bidirectional mode, it would be evident that there is no need for coercion to accomplish the objectives of this education, at every stage. This would be so were we in fact to ensure the appropriateness of the delivery mode, on the one hand, and of the details of the delivery itself being appropriate to the particular individual contextually, on the other. Thus, the nature of the delivery of education in whatever mode is crucial to its success, which suggests the need for contextualizing the delivery even in a particular based on the peculiarities of the health jurisdiction in question. The point here is that of irrelevance of the legitimacy of education given the relevance of the delivery mode within the general framework of the simplistic/intricate dyadic. This underscores similar operations at a more generic level of the democratic principles that we would employ, based on the appropriate inculcation of, and acquiescence to education, in the processes crucial to our health systems moving forward. Thus, we see, yet another dimension of education in health, still within the context of the achievement of the DHDO, of its role in fostering the establishment and evolution of democratic principles, and institutions, necessary for our health systems to move forward. For example, and in relation to the central position of the healthcare consumer in the healthcare delivery enterprise, such institutions, established would ensure the accountability and transparency in health systems operations that would promote public confidence in the operations necessary for their success. Furthermore, they would offer, in case such attributes are lacking, the healthcare consumer the choice of exit, for example, which is again crucial to such flawed health systems reorienting themselves, which is necessary to ensure the forward motion of the health systems in question. This issue also underscores the point made earlier about the individual/community dyadic, the dissatisfaction of the individual resulting in an exit from that health system for example, an important determinant of the health system's survival. In say in a privately funded health system arrangement, such loss of patronage could make that health system, say a hospital, non-viable economically any longer, which in fact could also happen in a publicly funded health system, for slightly different but related reasons. Such a health system, would therefore not be able to serve the community it was there to serve, to avert which situation, would therefore mobilize the community to action to rectify the flaw, even though it started with the dissatisfaction of an individual healthcare consumer. The chances of such mobilized action being possible at all depends on the community being well informed about relevant issues, hence the role of the appropriate education in this regard. This, coupled with the resulting likelihood of the appropriate democratic avenues in place, would result in the community also able to actually, sanction the demise of the particular health establishment in question if impossible to salvage it, exiting to another. Thus, we see education playing the dual role of instilling in the healthcare consumer the knowledge required to activate the democratic principles indispensable to the health system moving forward, also as it ensures that the health system inevitably responds to the requirements of not just the centrally-positioned healthcare consumer, but also its survival needs. In effect, education becomes the dominant driver in the achievement of the dual healthcare delivery objectives (DHDO).

The role of education in health is indeed, multiple, and complex, but they interlock at different levels to result in the results that our interventions at these different levels have occasioned. It is for this reason that we need to be conversant with the importance of our role in the entire endeavor of healthcare delivery, and in particular, that of education in ensuring its forward motion. As we earlier noted, this lack of awareness seems to be holding many health systems back worldwide, a situation none could afford, and one that could potentially set health systems back significantly. Indeed, it could set the entire country in which they operate back considering the importance of health for the economy. Here again, it is relatively easy to see how such compromised health systems could by becoming even costlier to run due to increasing disease prevalence, could eat substantially into the country's economic resources, compromising its ability to deliver other essential services. It is also not difficult to see how this situation would compromise the country's economic productivity, adversely affecting its businesses and industries, making them less competitive, in an increasingly competitive global marketplace. Thus by not having the appropriate concept of the key roles of education in healthcare delivery, we would not just be putting the health system in jeopardy we might actually be compromising the very survival of our country. Again, as we earlier noted, part of conceptualizing education appropriately involves revisiting its fundamentals, and in particular, reorienting healthcare delivery based on the correct formulations of the applicability of these fundamentals to healthcare delivery. An example of such formulations is that of the recognition of the value of both simplistic and intricate educational approaches in every health jurisdiction. We also need to emphasize the significance for health, of all healthcare stakeholders embracing the technologies that would facilitate the achievement of our educational goals, and this does not necessarily mean only in the developed countries. As we noted earlier, developing countries are also utilizing these technologies, in particular, the cellular phone, and the potential of such widespread use for targeted and contextualized health information/news delivery is doubtless immense even in such countries. Thus, the idea of elucidating the fundamentals of the role of education in healthcare delivery should not stop with just knowledge acquisition, but should proceed to the next stage, which is its app ropriate utilization. One approach to such appropriate utilization for example is again in conceptualizing healthcare delivery in public health preventive terms, namely via primary, secondary, and tertiary prevention of diseases. Primary prevention being the prevention of disease onset in the first place, secondary prevention, its prompt diagnosis and treatment, and tertiary prevention, that of its complications, including the establishment of appropriate rehabilitation programs to minimize their devastating effects, assumes key education elements. Again, part of this approach and its successful implementation is the recognition of the need for its facilitation, and the adoption of the technologies that could enable us so to do. In other words, it is not enough to recognize the need for health education in primary prevention for example, as the accomplishments of any education initiatives depend more on its delivery, which brings forth the need for re-conceptualizing the hitherto simplistic/intricate educational approaches, which we mentioned earlier. The reported findings in studies of the 'shock' tactics of placing vivid pictures of the pathologies resulting from cigarette smoking on cigarette packs to dissuade smokers, is instructive in this regard. In the U.S, for example, cigarette warnings are verbal and offer legally adequate information, whereas in Canada, for example, they vivid, even gruesome, placing which on cigarette packs in the U.S., one study found would be more effective than current verbal messages and incur less 'Tobacco Control Program (TCP)' funds[2]. Another study, published on February 06, 2007 in the American Journal of Preventive Medicine, a four-year study that examined differences in warnings on cigarette packs, and their effects on smokers in Canada, the U.K., Australia and the U.S., found that those vivid images are not just effective in changing smoking behaviors, indeed, more so, the more graphic[3]. here again, we see the coalescence of the simplistic/intricate dyadic, that one does not need to have complex didactic instructions to appreciate the health message in a picture, quite evident, which by extension suggests the potential for the effectiveness of this approach also in less developed countries, at least in those parts where didactic education is lacking. This vivid display of the ill effects of smoking could therefore not necessarily appear only on cigarette packs in countries, both developed and developing. Indeed, considering the point made earlier regarding the leapfrog into mobile communication technologies in many countries in the developing world, including in those parts with little if any opportunities for didactic education, these technologies would be appropriate delivery portals for such images, and indeed, other health education initiative, appropriate to the contexts of particular health jurisdictions. The potential for the use of these technologies not just in developed, but also in developing countries, therefore is indicative of the benefits accruable from the re-conceptualizing not just education, but its role in healthcare delivery, which we have thus far discussed. It also highlights the significance to the entire exercise of the review of every aspect of education in its elemental and other forms in other to gain full insight into the tasks that confront us in maximizing the potential of education in moving healthcare delivery forward. In secondary prevention, for example, it is important for the healthcare consumer to appreciate the need to seek prompt professional help for the treatment when ill. That the healthcare consumer has the most current health information that would facilitate the recognition of illnesses is crucial to taking this step in many instances to prevent in some cases, even fatalities. Should we then not encourage the acquisition of such information by healthcare providers, and would the widespread diffusion of healthcare information and communication technologies (healthcare ICT) not help facilitate this acquisition? Part of our initiatives in education should therefore focus on promoting the pervasive implementation of these technologies among all healthcare stakeholders. There is no doubt for example that including the healthcare consumer in the electronic health records (EHR) information loop is indispensable to maximizing in full, the benefits of these technologies, with free flow of information between doctors and their patients enabled, as between doctors and other healthcare professionals, such health information sharing vital to improved patient care. Education therefore is not just important to healthcare delivery its modus operandi will continue to need upgrading in light of the frenetic pace, some would contend, of technological progress, and indeed, of progress in medicine, with its direct and indirect influence of progress in healthcare information and communications technologies, and indeed, in technology in general. Thus, these technologies straddle progress in education and health and influence developments in both that in turn influence those in each other. Doubtless, we could hardly benefit from either without the sort of exercise we have discussed here that would elicit various aspects of the education/health dyadic in ways congruent with changes in both public expectations of health services delivery, and with pressure from different other directions including in non-health domains on health systems to perform more efficiently and cost-effectively. To give another example from the prevention paradigm, for example, the enormous costs of the consequences both in the short and long terms of chronic diseases for examples we could minimize, even if we failed to prevent these consequences or even the illnesses in the first place, or the illnesses from becoming chronic. Doing so however, would again, in some cases require investments in a variety of resources, including healthcare information and communication technologies that could for example in a post-stroke patient, prevent falls that would require additional and costly surgical interventions, possibly, not to mention the psychological and physical distress to the individual concerned and their families. The point here is the recognition of the many factors and at the different levels that are significant in our considerations of the education/health dyadic. It is important also to know that we have control over many of the processes and issues involved in the outcome of this dyadic. We should also know that not recognizing and taking the appropriate actions on them would result in at best slowing the motion of healthcare delivery in our health jurisdiction, or in fact, and worse, making it wobble on the spot, or even slide backward.

Healthcare is going to be a key issue in the years to come in many, if not all

countries. The role of education in healthcare delivery will become increasingly more pervasive and complex, and will not just encompass disease prevention, but also include health promotion, sustenance, and restoration more than ever before. The increasing focus of health and education on these and other issues would also question the adequacy of prevailing paradigms in both domains, which would therefore need ongoing reviews and reformulations, with significant policy implications. It is therefore important that we adopt a different mindset, in a manner of speaking to these issues than we currently do, the accentuation of which point in essence is the goal of the discussion here. As we have also emphasized, a key aspect of the success of whatever initiatives we embark upon is the centrality of the healthcare consumer, the individual that the health services we aim to improve serve. This underlines the need for education initiatives to be cognizant of the individual, hence designed to remedy the information asymmetry noted to obtain in the particular instance. Thus, it matters not whether we adopt simplistic or intricate approaches, that we would need in many instances to adopt both actually likelier than not, the important thing being the delivery of effective materials to achieve stated educational goals. This assumes that the stated goals would also be contextual as the needs of different health jurisdictions would probably vary. Indeed, each jurisdiction, as part of the exercise aimed at determining what those needs are should engage in process cycle analyses, processes involving decomposition and exposition, with the revelation along the way of additional issues and processes, and the mechanisms for their modifications, including exclusion if necessary of certain of them, on an ongoing basis. The ongoing nature of this exercise is important to stress considering that changes to the health system and its components are also ongoing, failure to accommodate which changes result in the entire health system or some of its parts becoming defective, and inadequate to cope with the demands of achieving the dual healthcare delivery objectives (DHDO) mentioned earlier. Thus, the health system is inherently unstable, and imperfect, and indeed, could never be perfect on this account, hence the need for instituting the mechanisms for such continuous evaluation process. This is not just for determining the education needs in the health system, but also to ensure that the system as a whole moves ever closer to perfection, that is, that the system engages, always, in the forward motion. Our efforts to appreciate in full the complexity of the relations between education and health are therefore, likely to involve a panoramic swing across the healthcare delivery enterprise and the resulting insight, likely to result in the profound changes that any health system would need to make on a continuous basis to survive, let alone thrive in the years ahead. This complexity is also going to reflect the evolution in a variety of domains relevant to that of the concept of education, an extension of the simplistic/intricate debate with if the phenomenon for example, we see shape up before our very eyes on the Internet termed social-networking, which websites such as MySpace and Facebook, popularized. It has in fact moved on to the next phase, into what some call social bookmarking or social news, exemplified by websites such as Digg.com, Reddit.com, Del.icio.us, Newsvine.com, and StumbleUpon.com. In this next phase, with readers able to vote for one another's stories and articles, which gain or do not gain prominence, with implications not just for advertising, trend identification, and enhancement of a company's products and services, but also for opinion formation, including on health issues. We see therefore, another potential dimension of education that could influence health and fitness practices, for example, predicated on the widespread use of healthcare information and communication technologies, in this instance the Internet. The implications for the accuracy of health information voted for, perhaps pushed by unscrupulous firms raises significant concerns, similar concerns already emerging in this domain as accusations of advertisers and marketers paying subscribers to these sites to vote for certain articles and stories have emerged, with the operators of the sites taking measures to plug potential avenues for such abuses. This also underscores the need for eclecticism in education and the applications of this diversity in approach to such fields as healthcare delivery, the point we made earlier about the simplistic/intricate dichotomy being outmoded, the use of both, and as we have also argued, even other approaches the direction education in health ought to go. The undercurrent of the need for this eclectic approach reflects the very nature of the evolution of human affairs, which healthcare delivery, and indeed, the influence on it of education, cannot ignore. In other words, there is certain inevitability in motion as we have noted that we could however influence, by our actions or inactions, for that matter, which determines what happens, not just to our health systems, but as they operate within the larger systems structure, to the entirety of our lives as humans. Education and health therefore, are merely vehicles, and there are many others, via which we traverse the spectrum of activities that contribute to which direction, and what eventually happens to the entire whole. In this more profound sense therefore, education becomes not just important, but crucial, to an equally critical healthcare delivery enterprise, both working in tandem to move humanity forward, if indeed, we made it so. The point here is that what happens to our health systems, and the role that education plays in what happens, depends in the main on what we do. What we do on the other hand depends on how we perceive what we should do. This is why the appropriate perception is a crucial first step in doing the right thing, which again underscores the need for education, indeed, and its appropriate perception, in ensuring our health systems move forward. It is important to have a reorientation in a manner of speaking therefore, of our approaches to education in the first place, for it to contribute the way it should to moving healthcare delivery forward. In the broader scheme of things, an appreciation of the very nature of the goals that we want to achieve individually and collectively is also crucial, as this in fact, would constitute a key driver of the actions that we need to take to achieve those goals. Here again, and as we have also noted, we need to discard entrenched notions on these goals, and be open to novel ways of conceptualizing them. It is redundant for example, to predicate the motion of our health system on its financing model, recognizing, as we should that it matters little if financed by public or private funds, whether we should commit to the delivery of qualitative health services efficiently and cost-effectively. In any case, again considering the key roles that healthcare ICT would play in the evolution of both education and health that we have emphasized in this discussion, both financing models would inevitably dovetail along identical dimensions, given that the widespread diffusion of these technologies materialize. Now we say given, actually surreptitiously as it is indeed, unlikely it would not be so. In other words, both publicly funded and privately funded health systems would increasingly realize the need for them to subscribe to the need to recognize the persistence of scarcity and to allocate and utilize resources prudently. We say increasingly because, and here is again, the beauty, so to say of the contribution of education, the expectations of the healthcare consumer of his or her health services could only become increasingly sophisticated and complex. That health systems would have to become more efficient and cost-effective to meet such increasingly suave healthcare delivery tastes is not contestable, nor is it that they, regardless of the funding model, would unlikely ignore, the potential contributions of healthcare ICT in helping them achieve these goals. These issues are going to loom larger over the coming years, and health systems should indeed, start to confront and address them from now, to avoid the possible adverse consequences of delays in not so doing on the motion of not just healthcare delivery, as we elaborated earlier, but in fact also on the entirety of our systems. Our discussion has highlighted the interplay of factors that we can no longer ignore if we were to move our health systems forward. These factors would become increasingly complex and more difficult to untangle if we did not start doing from now on. It is epiphenomena that it ongoing and those we need to understand their operations, which in fact that we could see their consequences, should make much easier. It is however, one thing to see the consequences all around but quite another to take the necessary measures to understand the phenomena as they pile one atop the other in a never-ending cascade of change of which we must ask ourselves if all we could is play catch-up. As we have repeatedly observed in this discussion, this is hardly in keeping with the accumulation of knowledge that we could ballyhoo, what could apparently be the problem perhaps is an oversight on our part, of the need for this veritable knowledge-base to also evolve in their applications to the movement of all the constituent processes of our systems. Considering the importance of healthcare delivery to the realization of our individual and collective objectives to survive, it is doubtful how much longer we could continue to ignore for example, the crucial role that healthcare information and communication technologies could play in our achievement of this goal. Indeed, we would have little to gain continuing to deploy the means that research evidence shows could help us achieve our goals, even outside the technology domain. The point then is that we should begin to appreciate the multiplicity of the factors crucial to our achieving our goals, and how best we could harness the resources available to us, and in fact develop new ones in addressing these many issues and in ensuring that we achieve our stated goals.

References

1. Available at: http://blogs.educationau.edu.au/nlothian/2006/12/13/taxonomy-directed-folksonomies/ Accessed on January 28, 2007

2. Ashish N., Fereydoun A, H arvey C. Comparison of current U.S and Canadian cigarette pack warnings. International Quarterly of Community Health Education. Volume 24, Number 1, / 2005-2006

3. Available at:
http://bodyandhealth.canada.com/channel_health_news_details.asp?news_id=11 681&news_channel_id=131&channel_id=131&relation_id=11576 Accessed on February 10, 2007

What has the Environment to do with Health?

A car battery recycling plant produced, when it rained, a haze that enveloped

Paraíso de Dios, God's Paradise, but years after its relocation, children are still born with high blood lead levels. This neighborhood in Bajos de Haina, 20 km west of the Dominican Republic capital, made the 2006 ten most-polluted list of the Blacksmith Institute based in New York[1]. Indeed, a study conducted in 2005 by the Dominican Republic Academy of Sciences reported that 93 percent of health consultations in Bajos de Haina, the country's industrial hub since the

1970s with over a hundred assorted industries, including its oil refinery, were 93%, 83%, 69%, and 68%, respectively for asthma, bronchitis, flu symptoms, and acute diarrhea[2]. Should we worry about this or the exponential increase in Latin America, for example, of mobile telephony, with the region bereft of coherent policies on handling used/outmoded and cellular telephones some of whose constituents, for example, the batteries could have levels of metals including cadmium, lead, nickel and mercury oxide, toxic to the environment and to health[2]? Should the region, and indeed, others, for example, in Africa, where there is also a sharp increase in cellular phone subscribers, not be initiating re-use, and recycling programs for not just cellular phones, but electronic wastes in general, or should they not? What role could the companies that manufacture these products play in such programs, and should there be legislation in place to ensure that they play such roles and if not how else could we ensure that they do? Still in Latin America, what should we say of the activities in the early 1980s at the climax of the gold rush of the garimpeiros, small-scale, self-employed gold diggers of Serra Pelada, deep in the Amazon in Brazil, vis-à-vis the then state-owned firm, Vale do Rio Doce (CVRD)? What should we say of the potential of regulations to prevent the deforestation and water pollution from the mercury used in mining operations, resulting from these activities, and which indeed, persist, with continuing discoveries of new El Dorados in the country? May be these issues bear little relevance to the much taunted, 'reducing greenhouse gas emissions,' that not even the purveyors of the annual jamborees of United Nations climate negotiations tire to ballyhoo, perhaps if the growth in emissions being slower, among member nations represents some form of reduction, could count for progress. One wonders what then this makes of the conclusions reached recently by the Intergovernmental Panel on Climate Change (IPCC) that the net effect of human activity since 1750 has been to warm up the globe, and that this is ongoing, temperatures projected to increase by 1.8-4C (3.2-7.2F) by the end of the century, sea levels, by 28-43cm₃. Now that IPCC is at least 90% certain that human emissions of greenhouse gases not natural variations are warming the planet's surface, versus its 61% certainty in its 2001 report, would we accept slowing emissions' growth or demand no growth, or indeed, accept nothing short of reducing the emissions drastically altogether? With the position of the IPCC on the role of human activity in generating these emissions having changed from 'likely' in 2001 to 'certain' in 2007, what prospects does this portend for a similar, even if incremental positive change in attitude of all concerned? Thus, that changes in the environment, brought on by human activity could result in adverse health consequences has struck the appropriate chord so to speak among 'all concerned' is in fact moot. It is not difficult for the garimpeiro to adduce reasons for digging massive holes in the earth in a desperate search for deposits of alluvial gold, when a minute quantity of the precious metal could earn a monthly wage, never mind what multiples of which the resulting health problems would cost to cure, if at all possible. As the examples above show, that economic considerations drive the human activities that increase emissions levels is just as applicable to the corporate as it is to the individual. Indeed, this issue is at the core of the pervasive, seemingly lackadaisical attitude toward climate change evident all around us. It is one, which we need to rethink in very fundamental ways. This would likely enable us appreciate fully, hence be liable to act speedily on, the ramifications for us, paradoxically in those very economic terms, to avert the consequences we purport, albeit indirectly through our studied inaction, or muted action, of our activities regarding greenhouse emissions. We need to start by acknowledging the essential role of all concerned in the process, that this is not just a matter of businesses through their manufacturing plants, and other activities, polluting everywhere and everything, or of governments doing little to agree on and take measures to stop them doing so. Every one of us has a stake in the matter, which we must accept, and we must take ownership of our responsibility in whatever direction in this regard, on the increase or decline in the emissions. This singular act should translate into the duty to act that we expect of not just one another, but also of businesses and governments. In other words, we would be morally justified to demand action from others, at whatever level only if we took that step of acknowledging ownership of the issues involved and responsibility for actions to reduce the emissions. There is an urgent need for a Rawlian 'veil of ignorance' at this critical 'original' state to kick-start this process, which has seemingly stalled, and would likely remain so, without concerted and determined efforts to accept responsibility for our stakes in this all-important issue. It is evident that there is gathering of the momentum, and a critical mass is imminent where collective action could redirect motion, but at what pace, and in which direction, of the emission reduction dimension, remains conjectural, again for the very reason of the economic considerations mentioned earlier holding sway at virtually all levels of human operations. It is therefore likely that the green movement would have increasing say, but would they have enough to change the direction of government on these issues in the key countries, which incidentally, do not currently seem inclined to do anything dramatic to change their directions on emissions, again mostly based on economic considerations. We are therefore likely to see a perpetuation of the very activities that we now know amount to 'mass, even if slow suicide' by us all. Traversing the different domains of these activities, are economic considerations, which incidentally, and as noted earlier, would become obvious in our discussion here, as antithetical to the goals they aim to achieve. To illustrate the absurdity of some of the arguments of the protagonist of this perspective, some contend that we need economic prosperity, which reducing greenhouse emissions would compromise, whereas which we could deploy in tackling whatever problems these emissions pose down the road. Such positions underline the need for the exercise that we need to conduct in a fuller appreciation of the issues at stake beyond mere intellectualizing, even if it provided the heuristics for such epiphany. In the first place, the economy is about transactions among humans, at least for now. Even when and if humanoids appear, transactions imply the pursuit of benefit by either party. This fundamental principle again highlights the points made by John Rawls of the need for a level playing field. It would therefore be easier for everyone to conceptualize the validity of the consensus we reach on issues, including the need to cut greenhouse emissions. The point in fact is that of the doubt of the potential for eliminating the graft in some quarters that make a mockery of the professed desire cloaked in veneer for the reduction in the emissions, or in general of the adverse consequences of the exploitation of the resources natural and otherwise that result in these emissions, otherwise. Thus, the prevalence of the preferred process of such extraction of the sham could only be a matter of time, given the efficient operations of our democracies, which continue to progress regardless. Rawls 'justice as fairness' therefore is indeed, an inevitable process, regardless of the 'veil.' The 'fairness' lies in the relentless efforts by all concerned for the establishments of the appropriate and relevant institutions even in established democracies suited to our contemporary times, the acceleration of which process is the real practical issue that confronts us and could determine how fast we slow down, if not eliminate this unwitting tendency toward 'mass suicide' mentioned earlier. In other words, the state of affairs could only go in three key directions, the directions in between which would eventually align with one of which. These directions are forward, backward, or wobbling on a spot. Indeed, even unlikely it is that one could wobble one a spot eternally without dissipating, at least from the perspective of the forward motion being incrementally survivalist, and the backward, moribund. Thus, regardless of the differentials in individual endowments, the cumulative tendency of motion is forward, not backward, although this latter position, appears tenable, albeit paradoxical, given the accumulation of knowledge, hence civilization that we have. It is excusable, and some might put this forward, that the pattern we deem moribund, is a mere disruption of the incremental 'philosophic value' of this millennia of accrued insight, that the train of knowledge would, so to say, redirect itself, obscuring the deviant path we now tread regarding climate change. Besides the question of the ease in so doing and in particular in obscuring the potential adverse consequences thereof, that we might not be fully cognizant of the fundamental roots of the issues involved might make such a redirection a dream. In other words, we might in fact be heading for the apocalypse, worse still because of economic considerations we would have apparently misconfigured.

The institutions that would strengthen our resolve to redirect our motion for

examples, those that ensure accountability, and the efficient and cost-effective operations of the transactions referred to above, would create the enabling environment to weed graft, for example, which would ensure the pursuant of the objectives of resource utilization without increasing greenhouse emissions, genuinely. Here again, the Rawlian, veil would be this deep appreciation of the fundamental issues that enable us work tirelessly to establish such institutions in the first place. It is also that which creates an 'original' position now, as we realize the significance of such establishments and other actions that we take to make our lives and societies more efficient and qualitative, in making us achieve not only our economic goals, but also all else. It is an interesting parody the paths of the previous great civilizations that lost direction, the championed emergent direction, relic of that, hitherto lost, the potential for accretion on which latter, clearly salvageable preceding the demise. Even the delay in forward motion that could ensue not fully appreciating the fundamentals could result in this travesty, which differentially among nations could manifest in an initial wobbling, which the seeming economic prosperity that would eventually turn out to be a farce would spawn, but which with appropriate measures taken to redirect, the motion would, in time, help reverse. This implies therefore that the only true direction of economic prosperity is the forward direction, and one that discountenances the need for us to avert the other two potential directions, and to actually, do so, flawed. That it is would emerge as we expose these fundamental issues in our discussion, in particular as we synthesize the various dimensions of these fundamentals, which with their tendency to seemingly operate independently obfuscate that to do so in tandem, both operational proclivities, nonetheless crucial to the eventual prospects of moving the motion forward. It is therefore likely for most to concur that the environment influences health either way, positively or negatively, although it might not be so evident in all cases, and indeed, not mention the influence on the other hand of the effect of the influence of the environment on health, on all other aspects of our lives, including on the economy. These other adjunct effects might in fact be seemingly operating not just independently but sometimes antagonistic to one another. This competitive situation coincides in collaboration, eventually, for the full realization of the objectives of either. That this in turn would be operational is our thesis here, with our for example, aligning in the direction of curtailing and eliminating the greenhouse-emission menace, the real issue being facilitating this process, given the delay in initiating actions in this direction thus far, which would persist not rethinking the issues, as the exposition of their fundamental roots herein demands. It is thus ominous that we should disregard the significance of the need for preserving the environment as sine qua non for so doing for health as the example of the gold diggers mentioned above clearly shows. On the other hand, that we should create an enabling situation to promote the health of our peoples to ensure that they do not degrade the environment and create additional health problems on top of that is not just positive but necessary. It thus follows that whereas we profess to want to avert the latter and pay little attention to the former, that we would seem inclined if at all, to a pristine milieu would be likelier than being indeed so. Our cacophony would drown genuine efforts in the end blurring entrenched divisions, the issues emergent from which chaos, even sorer. We would all lose in the end from the failure for whatever reason to conceptualize the fundamentals of the health-environment dyadic when in fact we could have won. Yes, it is quite realistic to expect us to achieve our stated objectives of eliminating the emissions given we grasped these fundamentals, the irony in not so doing evident in the simplicity of the outcome measures it dictates, for example, the acquiescence by all of the potential for our health systems embracing the technologies that could help improve healthcare delivery. This might appear starker considering the assertion recently by U.S. national health IT coordinator David Brailer in a *Health Affairs* interview in mid-February 2007[4], that these technologies could reduce healthcare spending up to 50 percent, but only after their widespread adoption for at least a decade. This underscores the point made earlier about the potential adverse consequences of delays in moving motion forward. In other words, a key aspect of our efforts in preserving the environment involves expediting actions, that is, whatever actions we deem appropriate in achieving this goal cannot wait. This principle of expediting actions applies to other aspects of our affairs, including not just health and the environment. The point has to do with the concept of motion itself and the changes that come with it. These changes influence our processes and we need to respond to these influences promptly or else they accrue, and become more complicated, and indeed, costlier to attune to the status quo, which itself is changing. If we needed ten years of full healthcare ICT implementation to be able to cut health spending in half, delaying the implementation would obviously prolong the realization of this pecuniary goal. Brailer noted that studies of other U.S. industries that have automated on a large scale, for examples, retail, banking, manufacturing, food, and insurance industries, indicated it took so long after the most of the players automated for its full benefits to show. That most solo and small doctors' practices, safety-net clinics, and practices in remote, rural, and underserved areas in the U.S are not automated is instructive in this regard. Considered contextually with the country's health spending projected in 2006 at $2.1 trillion, 16% of its gross domestic product (GDP) and projected to double over the next decade from current levels to reach $4.1 trillion, which would represent about twenty cents of every dollar spent, the implications of not grasping the fundamentals become even more vivids. The economists, and actuaries from the Office of the Actuary at the Centers for Medicare and Medicaid Services (CMS) in their annual forecasting report, also forecast the average annual health spending growth would remain steady at 6.9% between 2006 and 2016, even, fall a bit from 6.9% in 2005 to 6.8% in 2006, the fourth consecutive spending-lull year. At the end of the day, which perhaps explains the debate in Congress of a Bush administration proposal to cut $26 billion from Medicaid spending over the next five years, we would expectedly worry about the country's health spending. Yet, a recent research stresses the need instead of worrying about it to focus on fundamental programs reform to purge interstate variations in benefits and assist the states in managing increasing health costs[6]. Recently too, researchers argued that the projected fall in employer-sponsored insurance, and seniors' long-term care needs regardless, average Medicaid spending as a share of national health spending would be 16.6% between 2006 and 2025, same, 16.5% as in 2005, then increase slowly to 19.0% by 2045[7], increases that projected government revenues growth would be large enough to sustain. These studies, all point toward the possibilities of health services provision to the country's underprivileged, and indeed, to all, if it took the necessary measures to cut costs where they really ought to be. Given that we accept these facts and take these measures, we would then, at least in theory be able to achieve our goal of providing that enabling environment that would obviate the need for drastic measures to assure sustenance, which would not only help preserve the environment but also prevent additional health problems. As tenuous as this link between a healthy individual and pristine environment might appear, it is at the core of the success, or failure of any effort to preserve the environment, and it underscores the futility in not grasping the fundamentals mentioned earlier in fact pursuing this goal. It also transitions our conceptualizations across levels and explains the need for the companies, for example involved in the gold digging also to appreciate this futility. It brings to the fore again, our contention also earlier of the coalescence, necessarily of the forces of competition into collaboration, at once exigent, and imperative, which all entrenched positions must adopt. In other words, it is in the interests of the business sector to have a viable labor base, one comprising healthy motivated persons ready to drive their respective visions toward their goals.

It is teasing out this intricate link between health and the economy that would

reveal that between health and the environment in its entirety, and the counter-productiveness of economic considerations as sole reasons for not ensuring for example that we reduce, and indeed, eliminate the emissions. We want to see the healthy individual with a decent job unlikely keen to engage in another that would expose him or her to toxins, for example. In other words, the fundamentals involved with creating the enabling environment for such a healthy state would include rectifying the information asymmetry required to be able to make such a crucial decision regarding one's health, among others. We also want to see companies operate more responsibly cognizant of the damage they would do to their prospects otherwise. Thus working from the basics would enable all parties appreciate the stakes involved in preserving the environment, in particular the potential to compromise not just individual health, but also that of the country's economy, and by extension, adversely influence the very economy on which the survival of all depend. Examples of the direct and even indirect adverse effects of the environment are legion, and in general, known, which begs the question regarding the need to know that the environment could damage health. Thus, it is not necessarily because we are not conscious of the detrimental effects to our health of the emissions is why some countries balk at the idea of controlling theirs. This emphasizes the need for all to engage in this exercise of trying to understand fully the ramifications of the consequences of these emissions. The question would no doubt arise in some quarters of the problems realizing such objectives across board, the answer to which the very exercise would reveal. In other words, the primary objective for example, of ensuring the provision of qualitative healthcare for all is quite different from the mechanics of healthcare provision, although the mechanics would determine the achievement or otherwise of the primary objective. The accomplishment of the particular objectives of healthcare delivery in health jurisdictions would in effect be different, based on their peculiar local circumstances, although common to all health jurisdictions for example, would be the need to ensure that the healthcare consumer has sufficient information to be discerning regarding whatever decision taken on health matters. Each health jurisdiction would therefore need to appreciate the general and specific issues involved in our efforts to deliver on our promises both in the health and environment domains. This interplay of factors at the generic and specific levels is crucial for us to appreciate in our efforts to decipher the full impact of the environment-health dyadic. This is more so as it operates not just in each domain, but also as they interact to influence each other. Put differently, such appreciation is necessary for the realization of the goals we set out to achieve in either domain. It is thus the case that we would continue to wobble on the spot in most probability not so doing, creating by our own making the sort of delay mentioned above that could set us back perhaps even more than a decade in certain instances. Hence we would to avert such scenarios recognize the significance of wanting to see an individual not engage in activities that would degrade the environment, or increase emissions, creating the enabling milieu for that to happen. This would, in a particular jurisdiction say where the options for the sort of gold-digging exercise mentioned earlier exist involve, facilitating the creation of alternative employment opportunities, on the one hand, and the appropriate health services to operate in tandem, on the other. It is clear that we would be increasing the prospects of seeing individuals that would eschew jobs that could compromise their health even if they existed, as it is counterintuitive to be healthy and employed in a decent job, to opt for another that would jeopardize one's health while hardly paying more, even if it did. Thus, we see the potential influence on health of employment opportunities, and of both on the environment. We also start to see the concept of the fundamentals we have talked so much about emerge in earnest, the complexity of the essential elements germane to the interplay of health and the environment crucial as this elucidation unfolds. In other words, we cannot be talking about climate change in a vacuum, or for that matter, the need to preserve the environment ion general. Until we are able to tease out the elements and appreciate the importance of their interplay, we would be wasting precious time addressing the climate change and environment issues. Further to our argument about the potential changes an individual could undergo given the right circumstances, health delivery and employment opportunities, it is clear the role that businesses would play in this regard. In other words, another aspect at jurisdictional level would be to encourage the establishment of small and medium-sized businesses, since not all the big businesses could be everywhere, every time, besides even if they could. It would be equally clear to these businesses that an enlightened and healthy populace would be disinterested in such jobs that would jeopardize their health or would degrade the environment, hence would be unlikely to establish such jobs in the jurisdiction. This underscores the point made earlier about the coalescence of competitive forces, and the resultant benefits to all. It also underlines the need for rectifying information asymmetry and improving literacy levels, which would provide individuals with the necessary tools for rational decision-making on all matters, including those pertaining to health and employment. Thus, an important aspect of the mechanics mentioned earlier in, for example, ensuring the appreciation of the full ramifications of the emissions or of environmental degradation in general, across board, would be such efforts at rectifying information asymmetry. That this dialectical process would bear the desired results in the end is evident in the increasing demand by the consumer in many developed countries for automobiles that do not use fossil fuels, for example, those that are battery operated, and to which vehicle manufacturers are responding appropriately. Thus when we talked about jurisdictions encouraging businesses to establish operations in their areas, we did not say force them to do so, as it is evident from the above example of the potential for voluntary responsiveness by businesses to the demands, even for employment opportunities. In other words, it would not be too long before someone realizes the potential for the large pool of even particular labor in jurisdictions, as the case of India, and some other Asian countries where information technology companies have created businesses for new business models, with resounding success. The point here is that it is not always the case that businesses have the upper hand in determining what sort of businesses to establish. Indeed, they quite often strategize based on a variety of factors including the availability and cost of labor. In any case, even if local authorities do not dictate what businesses to establish, they could at least regulate them, and ensure for example that they do not degrade the environment in their operations, or put the health of the populace at risk. The turkey farm in Holton, Suffolk in the UK, where an outbreak of bird flu among the turkeys, announced on February 03, 2007, blamed at least in part on gulls carrying waste from the site, a nearby meat-processing part of the farm, exemplifies this points. There is no doubt local authorities would have to take measures to ensure establishment and compliance with standards that would avert potential health risks due to the operations of these businesses that they nonetheless need to attract to their communities. It would also be necessary for these businesses to ensure compliance with the measures, as it would be in their best interests to have a healthy labor force to employ, even not considering the morality of such compliance. In other words, it is in the economic interests of all parties to ensure that the environment is not toxic to individuals, via either heavy metals or virulent bugs, for examples. Part of the process of emphasizing these points to businesses is inherent in the nature of business itself, but the regulations mentioned above should focus on such enlightenment efforts, than on enforcement of measures the full ramifications of which the companies and their employees might not in fact appreciate. This is more so if not evident regarding their links to the companies' bottom-line, for example. Thus, the focus of rectifying information asymmetry should be multidirectional therefore, not just individuals, but all elements of society involved. This in fact highlights the point we made earlier about the counter-productive nature of not preserving the environment, the reasons for which mostly involve economic considerations. Thus, we would in fact be worsening our economic status in the end, not so doing. This could be due to the direct effects of climate and environmental changes on business operations, on the one hand, and to those of compromised health due to these changes, and indeed, to both on the other.

The workings of the mechanics of healthcare provision, and the primary

objectives, that set them in motion, become increasingly important therefore, as all the elements of society keen to preserve the environment progressively appreciate and accept the futility of the supremacy of economic considerations in their decisions on regarding the emissions for example. In other words, it becomes easier to formulate and implement policies at jurisdictional levels that would ensure the provision of qualitative health services accessible to all. The significance of the provision of these services would have become clear as would have been the need for initiatives to ensure the provision. We have seen thus far then, that the environment issue is more complicated than it seems on the surface and that to achieve the goal of preserving the environment, including preventing further damage to the climate by hydrocarbon emissions, is more than organizing periodic intergovernmental meetings or protest marches. We all have to be realistic about the fundamental measures necessary for us to appreciate and to take to achieve this goal and that these measures need to start now, as the longer we delay the actions required the more difficult achieving the goal would be and the longer it would take. These measures would result in individual and corporate actions, both crucial to the achievement of the goal. At the core of these measures as our discussion has shown is the need for the appropriate knowledge at different levels, which is critical for the achievement of the healthcare provision goals, for example, themselves crucial to the preservation of the environment. The fundamental overwhelming desire for the majority of persons to survive would be the driving force of the motorizing attributes of this core activity, in other words, the imperative underlying the concerted efforts that would evolve at different levels to achieve our goals of healthcare provision, and by extension, of environmental preservation. This underscores the point about the potential of these efforts to proceed without enforcements, so as the initial triggers, for example the appreciation of the fundamentals that we have discussed here, are operational. This is why we cannot afford to delay the initiation of these efforts, as we would have to initiate them anyway, and such delays could only complicate matters for us all. There are ongoing changes in biotic and abiotic, living and nonliving factors, respectively, to which we are exposed, and both groups of factors influence each other in a symbiotic dyadic, these ongoing changes, requiring us to adapt, which if we did not could create adversity that could make us moribund. Our ability to survive until now despite the sometimes-destructive effects of the abiotic factors such as temperature, light, water, and ionizing radiation, for examples, attests to our inherent desire to overcome odds to do so. This is also evident in our being able to surpass other biotic elements, and indeed, to control them, as it is our proclivity to damage the abiotic elements, evident of our indictment in the report of the Intergovernmental Panel on Climate Change (IPCC) announced in early February 2007[9], mentioned earlier. That the report noted that our activities caused global warming is instructive of the magnitude of the effects of actions over which we have control on our environment. It also underlines the urgency of the arguments we have put forward regarding the fundamentals that we all need to start to appreciate and now. This is more so as this report does not constitute entirely new knowledge, as also noted earlier. It is also significant that the report dated our activities that resulted in global warming back to the Little Ice Age (LIA) (1750); a period of cooling that took place after a warmer era termed by Climatologists, the medieval climate optimum. This is considering the varieties of developments in the human arena in the C18th including a number of major wars, the French Revolution, and the publication of seminal works by Adam Smith, David Hume, and Edmund Burke among others with profound influence on human affairs, not to mention the industrial and technological revolutions that have occurred since then. Is it any wonder then that John Ashton, the UK's climate change envoy remarked in September 2006 that we must consider human-induced climate change an urgent threat to national security and prosperity, and stressed the need to secure a stable climate at whatever cost, as not so doing would cost even more? Was he wrong in also noting that any government's first priority is providing the enabling milieu for security and prosperity in return for its citizens' taxes, and that climate change is p robably the gravest threat ever to this most basic of social contracts[10]? When on August, 28, 2005, New Orleans, a hitherto prosperous American city, after being hit by Hurricane Ka, became the exemplar of the horror nature could bestow on us in a developed country in recent times, we learnt first hand the need to pay to preserving the environment, or did we? Examples abound in other countries and regions of natural catastrophes experts attribute directly or indirectly to global warming as they do the potential devastation on economies of these natural disasters, if they indeed qualified as such. This is particularly so in third world countries whose economies struggle to stay afloat, the disruptions they cause, sometimes resulting in tribal conflicts, even wars, with serious implications for health and further economic devastation. Do we therefore not need to appreciate the fundamentals that we discussed here, for example, that would enable the appreciation by all of the need for soft, not hard power in getting everyone to commit to reducing and indeed, eliminating hydrocarbons emissions? Would it not help to appreciate the futility of military force in stopping a hurricane from touching land, or stemming a rising tide, or preventing glaciers melting? Should we also not adopt the same principles in addressing these issues at the individual and other levels as previously discussed here? Again the mechanics of operations at different levels would vary, and do not have to wait for the accomplishment of one another, so long as the framework for motorizing initiatives at different levels are in keeping with the overall goal. Governments for example would still need to negotiate the agreements that would facilitate initiatives at local jurisdictions to reduce emissions, for example, as efficiently and cost-effectively as current circumstances permit, while particular jurisdictions set in motion initiatives of their own, for examples, based on the premises discussed here. In other words, our efforts to reduce emissions, and preserve the environment must proceed apace, and within a general framework, such that the exercises engaged in as parts of our efforts to elucidate and appreciate fully the fundamentals mentioned earlier would be evident at all levels. Thus, we cannot gainsay the importance of this fundamental approach to addressing not just the environment issue, but also in its applications to the health domain and vice versa. A key aspect of the implementation of this approach is, as we have noted, education, which ought to start from an early age. Thus, we should start from now to inculcate in our youths the importance of the environment for the continued survival of humankind. This does not imply that we should only focus on the youths. In fact, we need to focus, as already noted, on all segments of society as we all participate, one way or another, in the economic activities upon which many of the considerations that current stifle efforts to reduce greenhouse gases for example, pivot. This was the point made about the need to rectify information asymmetry earlier on. Just as we should not delay in our focus on the youths, we should start our initiatives to highlight the need to preserve the environment among adults and in the corporate world now, or as soon as practicable. Perhaps such widespread enlightenment regarding these issues would someday provide us more viable answers than the current and controversial arguments for carbon pricing and trading, the emphasis on cost-effectiveness of which for example discountenances the 'human issues' inherent in carbon dumping.

References

1. Available at: http://www.ipsnews.net/news.asp?idnews=36323 Accessed on February 04, 2007

2. Available at: http://www.ipsnews.net/news.asp?idnews=34555 Accessed on February 04, 2007

3. Available at: http://news.bbc.co.uk/2/hi/science/nature/6321351.stm?ls Accessed on February 4, 2007

4. Available at: http://www.healthcareitnews.com/story.cms?id=6418 Accessed on February 23, 2007

5. Poisal, JA, Truffer, C, Smith, S, Sisko, A, Cowan, C, Keehan, S, Dickensheets, B, and National Health Expenditures Team, Health Spending Projections Through 2016: Modest Changes Obscure Part D's Impact, *Health Affairs* Web Exclusive, February 21, 2007
Available at:
http://content.healthaffairs.org/cgi/content/abstract/hlthaff.26.2.w242 Accessed on February 23, 2007

6. Holahan, J and Alan Weil. Toward Real Medicaid Reform [*Health Affairs* 26, no. 2 (2007): w254-w270 (published online 23 February 2007; 10.1377/hlthaff.26.2.w254)]
Available at:
http://content.healthaffairs.org/cgi/content/full/hlthaff.26.2.w254v1/DC1
Accessed on February 23, 2007

7. Kronick, R, and David Rousseau Is Medicaid Sustainable? Spending Projections For The Program's Second Forty Years [*Health Affairs* 26, no. 2 (2007): w271-w287 (published online 23 February 2007; 10.1377/hlthaff.26.2.w271)]
Available at:
http://content.healthaffairs.org/cgi/content/abstract/hlthaff.26.2.w271v1 Accessed on February 23, 2007

8. Available at: http://news.bbc.co.uk/2/hi/uk_news/4882824.stm
Accessed on February 23, 2007

9. Available at:
http://newsvote.bbc.co.uk/mpapps/pagetools/print/news.bbc.co.uk/2/hi/science/nature/6321351.stm Accessed on February 24, 2007

10. Available at:
http://newsvote.bbc.co.uk/mpapps/pagetools/print/news.bbc.co.uk/2/hi/science/nature/5323512.stm Accessed on February 24, 2007

Who needs drug companies?

When Pfizer, the world's foremost drug company announced on January 22,

2007 that it would reduce its workforce by 7,800, close a number of manufacturing and research locations, and revamp its business practices, it was not that industry observers did not anticipate these measures. This is so in particular considering the seemingly endless difficulties that the pharmaceutical industry faces in recent times. Increasing competition of cheaper generic drugs, setbacks in new product development, and what many consider lingering image problems emanating from various sources, plague the industry and hurt its bottom-line. That Pfizer announced it was laying off 2,200 only a month earlier, and slashed its American sales force by 20%, even if these layoffs still represented just 10% of the company's global workforce, is no doubt, nonetheless instructive of the state of affairs not just in Pfizer, but in the entire pharmaceutical industry. It is indeed, the exemplar of the fundamental rather than incremental evolution that the new chief executive officer of Pfizer termed imperative, and must happen now, which many would argue in fact, not just in the company, but also industry wide. With profit-making drugs losing patent protection in many of these firms, generics creeping in from all directions, new drug development not keeping pace, sales force operations bursting at the rims, literally, the resulting chaos likely to be counter-productive, regarding prescription rates by doctors, the need for reorganization is no doubt evident. Pfizer, for example, wants to reorganize its sales force, and its research and development (R&D) to concentrate on specific diseases, which begs the question which diseases, and what the consequences for healthcare would be, considering not just the pivotal role of the company in drug manufacturing, but were its competitors to follow suit. This raises fundamental issues that should concern us all regarding not just the future of the pharmaceutical industry, but also of healthcare delivery, not to mention its implications for many other domains, outside these two. Pfizer expects to save $1.5 billion to $2 billion in annual expenditures, in addition to the $4 billion planned cost reductions by 2008. Although the firm's stock fell by 1% with this latest announcement, closing at $26.95, and it announced 2006 fourth quarter earnings fall, excluding special items, to 43 cents a share, from 49 cents in the same period in 2005, it expects the measures to buoy its earnings even from the 2006 $48.4 billion figures for 2007/2008 by 6%-9%. These measures thus, paradoxically highlight the dilemma they pose, being on the one hand potential lifesavers, and on the other, potentially the exact opposite, conceptualized broadly the firm included. In other words, at what point would such measures be counter-productive to the firm's legitimate yearnings, given their ramifications, for the firm, the industry, and indeed, for the healthcare industry, on whose very survival the firm, and the pharmaceutical industry in general depends? Yet, it is moot that the firm needed to sit back and become moribund. The balance thus, between slide into oblivion and remaining relevant seems tenuous, to say the least, if not outright precarious. Yet, with the firm essentially impelling its erstwhile boss to early retirement could anyone misconstrue the potential rigor in the offing makeover the firm, the new boss pledging to review all of the firm's operations, for example? Yet, there are those in the industry skeptical of continuous downsizing being epiphany, not when it does not appear that humanoid operatives would work out new drug development any time soon, in particular capping R&D at $7.5 billion. Looking at what biotech firms' acquisition could do for a firm such as Pfizer, with its recent loss of patent protection over Zoloft and Zithromax resulting 70% 4th quarter sales decline conjures a quixotic in some, nirvana in others, the firm included, not also with patent protection loss imminent for Norvasc, which grossed $4.9 billion for the firm in 2006. This is not to mention its equally imminent patent protection loss over Lipitor, the most profitable drug globally, in about three years, more so with its much-anticipated replacement, torcetrapib jettisoned for safety reasons in December 2006. The point here is that it is exigent for the firm to embark on fundamental organizational changes, even involving a marked departure from its customary chemical-based drug manufacturing processes to the protein-based models typical of the biotech firms whose products it might license or which it might purchase outright, as incidentally some of its competitors also propose. The issues that such exigencies spawn constitute another focus that could be just as exigent to ponder. Could anyone fault Pfizer, whose even Lipitor sales, which increased 6% in 2006 at

$12.9 billion, dropped by 1% in the 2006 4th quarter to $3.34 billion, with the

emergence of generic competition to Zocor, for making fundamental

organizational changes? Would we on the other hand, expect to have

medications for just certain diseases for example, as pharmaceutical companies

streamline R&D, and focus on drugs that would ensure their survival? How

could we thus, justify not taking the necessary measures to ensure that we do not

face such a dilemma? The answers to these questions, all probably affirmative

pose even more disturbing questions. Such questions concern in particular, our

appreciation of the crucial issues at play, the way we should, that is, if not that

we absolutely do not, in the health and pharmaceutical industries, crucial to each

other's survival, and to that of the entirety of the system within whose context

the interplay manifests. That the issues culminating in the events occurring in the

pharmaceutical industry, for example the layoff by Pfizer of thousands of its

workers, have been brewing for years is instructive in this regard. Could we for

example have stemmed their outcomes that seem to indicate a potential

transition to another level of the elements operational in this and in fact related

industries, for example, the health industry? What could have been the direction

of events now had the industry's credibility crisis that the withdrawal over three

years ago by Merck of Vioxx sparked taken a slightly different turn, for example

regarding drug approval by the Food and Drug Administration (FDA), or

doctors whose prescription patterns dramatically changed, sometimes without

sufficient scientific backing? What could have happened had insurance firms for

example not also embraced as a result older less expensive, and generic

medications, arguing equivalent efficacy with brands? Have the lingering effects

of these developments now created the dilemma that not just the pharmaceutical

industry, but the health, insurance, and other related industries, and indeed, all healthcare stakeholders confront, and the solution to which we must all be part of producing? That we need to have safe and effective drugs is not in question. What we need to consider is whether we could afford to run the pharmaceutical industry aground in the process. Granted that not even the pharmaceutical industry is immune to the market vagaries, but we do need to appreciate fully the mechanics of the markets in which firms in this industry operate, given its significance for the health industry in particular, on whose efficient and effective operations, so much that society depends on rests. Is it for example okay to expect any drug to be risk-free, or any medication not to have side effects, and should therefore, not consider these in determining the fitness or otherwise of medications for human consumption, as opposed to eliminating every drug with side-effects, willy-nilly from the formulary? What could be the overall implications of cuts in research budgets for the efficacy and safety of medications anyway, not to mention for the development of a wider variety of drugs for different diseases? With the combined loss of an estimated $10 billion in annual sales from the loss of patent protection by three of the largest drug makers in the US alone, is it any wonder that these firms, which spend significantly on R&D, the industry on the whole, over $30 billion annually, are cutting back? What further could we say for the pressure on the pharmaceutical industry with Wall Street for example, unforgiving on top of all these, shares of many of the pharmaceutical companies doing poorly, versus those of biotech firms for example, which are performing quite well, in the main? Tension within the industry could only increase with drug reformulations and guerilla consumer advertising not working that well anymore, R&D budget cuts not creating the chances of new 'wonder' drugs, and insurance firms not impressed with the reformulated drugs, anyhow, witness the row over the benefits of Zmax, and Zithromax, which Pfizer introduced in 2005 and 1992, respectively. There is no doubt about the potential crisis of survival confronting the pharmaceutical industry, as there is none either about its significance for the health and related industries. The pharmaceutical industry needs to be cognizant of what some would consider the public cynicism it currently faces, the result, again, of developments over the years that we could arguably possibly stem if we paid sufficient attention to so doing. Thus, issues of transparency and accountability that could have cleared up the looming public distrust over issues that have strained public opinion of the industry over the years escaped our scrutiny. It is apposite to eschew blame for our inaction as the issue at hand requires the urgency that to indulge in finding scapegoats fails to recognize, and in so doing, also to establish even the critical framework within which to seek and implement solutions, a necessary first step. In other words, we should accept collective responsibility for not appreciating the fundamentals of the interplay of the many drivers of our health systems, to which such inaction amounts. Is it for example important for the lack of or delay in disclosure of the potential clinical trials' evidence of the increased risk of suicidality in young persons for example due to taking certain antidepressants, of the distinction between the aspirations of the individual and the community regarding health? Could it be the case that this distinction is even more so considering the controversy surrounding the subject even among researchers, even now?

That the risk to any individual weighed against the benefits to the community

of the introduction of a particular medication, or the potential for not disclosing fully its danger to an individual are profound issues that have connived, some would contend, to compromise the image of the pharmaceutical industry, among others, due to the inaction referred to earlier. Yet, it is against this background that many view the increased rigor with which the FDA for example, conducts its business of approving new drugs, which many would also argue contributed significantly to the dilemma also earlier mentioned. To begin to conceptualize the various issues to which we must attend to wriggle out of the dilemma then, is in itself an exercise in methodological rigor, involving what we could term process cycle analysis, an ongoing decomposition/exposition exercise that would peel, so to say, the layers of epiphenomena that conceal every other, regardless of how cryptic. This exercise in addition to the revelation of the causal issues of observed phenomena would also reveal the appropriate solutions to them. It is crucial to emphasize the exercise, which is multilevel and multidimensional, being important to determining the nature of the fundamental changes that we need to make not just to the pharmaceutical, but also the health industry, for both to survive, let alone thrive. In recognizing for example, that we have not reached anywhere near eliminating diseases, we would continue to need the pharmaceutical industry that the survival of the industry is in the interest of healthcare stakeholders is doubtless. There is also no doubt that the industry also needs the health industry to survive for that to happen, the sort of mutual inter-dependence that calls for a reorientation of our approaches to the pharmaceutical industry. This inter-dependence underscores the need for a thorough understanding of the processes involved in the effective operations of both industries, singly, and at their interfaces, which ongoing process cycle analyses could no doubt help tease out. Is it possible for example, that with such understanding of the elements of the disease prevention paradigm would emerge opportunities for pharmaceuticals suited to multilevel, prim ary, secondary, and tertiary prevention initiatives, with a different bent from the customary? Is it also possible therefore, that the pharmaceutical industry would in evolving in tandem with the health industry undergo significant paradigmatic shifts, which would ensure its survival in keeping with the changing times? There is no gainsaying the possibility of the causality of the fundamental frameworks of both the pharmaceutical and health industries dovetailing for the reorientation that we contend that the contemporary pharmaceutical zeitgeist probably needs to move the industry forward. The issue transcends an apologist tendency for the multibillion investment of the industry in R&D for example to a dispassionate explication of the requirements for its success in the prevailing circumstances vis-à-vis the future, an appreciation of which the interests shown for example, by many of the larger pharmaceutical companies in biotech companies in recent times suggest. It is also in this context that in addition to establishing the appropriate machinery for facilitating transparency and accountability alluded to earlier, we need to emphasize also the need to rectify the information asymmetry characteristic of not just the health, but also the pharmaceutical industry. This incidentally is not always necessarily to foster the interest of the consumer, as the potential for benefits to the industry of the recognition by the public for example of educating the consumer regarding the potential for significant side effects inherent in all medications, another crucial initiative to promote transparency, is doubtless. That, pharmaceutical firms, could also boost the industries image by engaging in social programs beneficial to large segments of society, and promoting the availability of affordable medications in particular to the financially-challenged and the uninsured, is not also in doubt. These and other issues could almost certainly significantly improve the prospects of survival for the pharmaceutical industry, the stability of the fundamental platform for further progress so created by many of these measures, an essential element for not just survival, but continued profitability, a crucial aspect of survival in its own right. On a more technical level, the industry also needs to address such issues as data exclusivity, whereby they maintain exclusive rights to over clinical and preclinical trial data, which some critics argue could compromise efforts to produce generic versions of life-saving drugs, hence public health[1]. An example of such drugs is the "flu drug" oseltamivir, and some contend that data exclusivity is already limiting patients' access to generic HIV drugs. Yet, pharmaceutical companies could argue that they spent enormous time and money on the preclinical and clinical trials that helped establish the safety, efficacy, and quality of their drugs before approval by regulatory authorities to market them. However, this means that the smaller drug companies that typically market the generics would need to repeat these trials to establish the safety and efficacy of their own products, generic versions of the same products on which these data already exist, due to data exclusivity, an exercise that many could ill-afford. This is not to mention the ethical issues involved in repeating clinical trials, such as withholding medications with established effectiveness from some in the control group, for example. This issue could make it unlikely for generic firms to scale ethical review boards' requirements, hence conduct such clinical trials, putting them in a bind, at least until the end of the data exclusivity period. The implications of this delay for competition and lowered prices are another matter and the recent introduction by US legislators in the House and Senate on February 14, 2007 that would allow FDA approval of 'comparable' and 'interchangeable' generic versions of biotech medications through an 'abbreviated' process[2], edifying. The Access to Life Saving Medicine Act of 2007 and similar legislation many would argue would help generic drugs makers who now lack a clear regulatory corridor for producing cheaper alternatives of biopharmaceutical drugs. However, firms that plan to market analogous generic versions of biotech drugs would need to prove that they have active ingredients 'similar' and same effects to those in brand-name versions, although the legislation would not specifically mandate them to conduct clinical trials in general the FDA able to demand trials as it deems fit in particular situations. With some arguing that, the bill would reduce the cost of biotech drugs that could cost $5,000 or more/month, save lives, and save Medicare up to $14 billion, and consumers/health insurers, up to $71 billion in a decade, opponents that the chemical composition of generics could never be the same as that of the biologics, the argument rages. Biologics, such as insulin and cancer drug Herceptin, are living cells-based, versus conventional drugs that are chemicals-based, and the FDA approves generic versions of the latter when they lose patent protection, unlike, at least until the bill passes, with biologics that they not authority to approve hence shielded from competition at least in part from generics. Importantly, it leaves open the question whether granting FDA the power to choose when to order clinical trials even in this instance is in the end a wise thing to do. This question is pertinent considering recent developments in Europe with the passing into law of legislation that cover biosimilar medicines in France on February 06, 2007. The legislation prevents biosimilar medicines, copies of original or 'innovator' biotechnology medicines, similar but not identical to the original product, hence termed 'biosimilar,' not 'biogenerics,' from being classed as generics. It also outlaws the automatic swapping of biological medicines, which underscores the centrality of the healthcare consumer, and by extension that of the doctor/patient dyadic crucial to effective care delivery. It affirms the EU legal definition of a "biosimilar" medicine, acknowledging that these novel products are unique and not classifiable as 'generics' as chemical compounds are, because of differences in the active biotechnological substances and manufacturing processes. Weighed against the findings, released on February 20, 2007 by Express Scripts[3] that, averagely biotech drugs, now 25% to 30% of prescription drug costs for companies, cost $71,600/year versus $1,200 for standard drugs, the question becomes even more complex. If, as the study noted, biotech medication costs would likely double to $90 billion in 2009, thrice as fast as customary drugs, the issue of generic copies of these drugs will unlikely go away anytime soon. Indeed, that of generics in general would continue to haunt the pharm aceutical industry for some time to come if it did not address the issues involved such as those mentioned above effectively. The pharmaceutical industry needs to come to some form of agreement with those that make generics on pricing, which is the main sticking point of this matter, in the interests of the healthcare consumer, and more importantly, of the pharmaceutical industry, and indeed, related ones, such as the biotech industry. That some of the major pharmaceutical firms are engaged in making generics should make reaching such an agreement a lot easier. The urgency that reaching such an agreement warrants relates to a number of developments in both the pharmaceutical and health industries, and indeed, beyond. For example in the US, subsequent to mounting public concern with health risks posed by approved drugs, the Food and Drug Administration (FDA) requested the Institute of Medicine (IOM) to organize an ad hoc committee of experts. The committee was to carry out an independent evaluation of the current system for appraising and ensuring drug safety post-marketing and recommend measures to improve risk assessment, surveillance, and the safe medications use.

The committee in its report, *The Future of Drug Safety: Promoting and Protecting*

the Health of the Public, reiterated the importance of the role of the FDA regarding the drug safety system, which sums up its activities and reviewed major aspects of the roles and potential contributions to the system of the pharmaceutical industry, among others. It stressed the perception crisis that has dented the credibility of FDA and that of the pharmaceutical industry, including the flaws in both regarding openness and accountability regarding drug safety, which latter among others constituted key recommendations by the committee. This underscores the point we made earlier that the pharmaceutical industry needs to have an image makeover that would reflect its attunement to public expectations, and highlight simultaneously, its significant role in the healthcare d elivery enterprise. It has first to appreciate the fact that this role is inherent in the expectations of the public of its health system on the one hand, and of its part in the health system meeting that expectation on the other. It must also acknowledge however, that its role derives from its strategic objectives, spelt out in its commitments to the very instruments of its being, whose interests and those of the public incidentally coincide rather than are opposites. Finally, it needs to be cognizant of its place in the economic scheme of things in its jurisdiction of operations primarily, and in fact, in consonance with those of the related industries on which its very existence also crucially depends. That these multidimensional commitments are crucial to underline represents the not complexity of the operations that the pharmaceutical must engage in given the peculiarities of our contemporary times to stay afloat. In other words, it is okay for the industry to churn out novel medications or to strategize on so doing most cost-effectively, perhaps, foraying into biologics even more. Nonetheless, it also has to market itself as well to the public, to maintain a presence much unlike prior, to present a new face of friendship and cooperation in achieving comm on rather than opposing goals. Thus, in the public acknowledging that it needs the pharmaceutical industry, the industry also has to recognize the importance of its public image to its very survival. Part of enhancing its public image involves eschewing any issues that could cast a shadow on its transparency although it is arguable if had the leverage in all instances so to do, as the example in the US of the provisions in the fiscal year 2008 budget proposal released President Bush in mid-February 2007 shows. This proposal would increase user fees paid to FDA, which some contend would actually give the industry excessive influence over the agencys. Given that the issue dates back to the 1992 Prescription Drug User Fee Act, that mandates pharmaceutical firms to pay user fees in exchange for reviews of new drugs in a year or less, the commotion might not have been so much were it just renewed as it is by Congress upon its expiration this year. However, the President's budget proposal would not only increase funds for FDA by $100 million, which is in keeping with the recommendations of the committee referred to above, but it also includes a substantial increase in user fees and the first fees, for brand-name and generic pharmaceutical companies, respectively. In the FDA budget, $2.1 billion, in other words, includes $444 million in user fees from industries the agency regulates, including $15.7 million in fees from generic drugs firms, the increases, government insists are necessary due to an increase in the number of applications received by the agency. It is arguable that these increases in user fees would limit the agency's ability to ensure drug safety especially as even the Pharmaceutical Research and Manufacturers of America's projection that drug companies would fund roughly 60% of the cost of the agency's reviews on drugs applications in 2008, versus about 40% a decade earlier, it considered high. Part of efforts at the makeover mentioned earlier should include the industry making this position public for example, a position that others, such as the Biotechnology Industry Organization endorse, which organization maintained that user fees should not fund more than half the budget for these reviews. There is also, what the Federal Trade Commission calls exclusion payment settlements, settlements in patent disputes that more and more include agreements to delay generic competition in exchange for payments from brand name to generic drug firms, to curb which practice the Senate Judiciary Committee on February 15, 2007, approved legislation (S 316). This legislation would bar such payments to delay introducing generics into the market, a practice that many argue confine competition at the consumers' expense, who are unable to purchase drugs at reduced prices, sometimes for years. No doubt, the industry would want to reconsider its views of this matter. Improving the pubic image of the industry is an integral part of it being able to accomplish its strategic objectives owed its shareholders, and in many ways underscores the convergence of these goals with those of the public, which unlikely as it might seem is essentially the case. That both the public and shareholders are humans for one indicates an inherent convergence of the right to life mentioned earlier, which by extension also makes implicit that of their respective interests in ensuring the economic progress of the jurisdiction in which they operate, in particular, their country. Thus, the industry has much to gain and hardly anything to lose taking the issue of making over its image seriously. Indeed, and in another dimension, such efforts would increasingly confer competitive edge on pharmaceutical companies in a milieu in which excellence is going to take a variety of forms besides the conventional. Thus, such companies would be better able to meet their mandates to the various stakeholders mentioned earlier, more expediently. Pharmaceutical companies would increasingly find that price wars alone would be inadequate to meet the ever-complex challenges that the industry would face in the years ahead, their multimodal sources, the health, insurance, government, consumer, and even within-industry issues that would need varying degrees of urgency to resolve, at play individually and in association combined in equally multimodal forms. What would be clear amid this chaos would be the permanence of the pharmaceutical industry, even if the final form were anything but permanent. In other words, there would indeed, be no final form as the industry of necessity evolves in tandem with related industries, in particular the health industry, molded itself by a variety of health and non-health related forces. It is unlikely that the pharmaceutical industry for example would be oblivious to the increasing role that genetic engineering would play in healthcare delivery, with clearer understanding of the genome potentially spawning profound paradigmatic shifts in practice, which might involve equally dramatic changes in the use of medications, and indeed, the types used. In other words, the pharmaceutical industry would need, a reorientation in their strategic intent, benchmarking not necessarily against external validators but cognizant of the need for the industry itself to achieve certain set standards. It needs, for example, attunement to the need for ongoing self-analysis occasioned by the recognition of changes being inevitable, and of the necessary disruptions to the status quo, that would result, being drivers of the appropriate responses. This would make it responsive and indeed, nimbly so, to the changes occurring in the health and related industry, the pace in the former at least, some would describe as frenetic. Considering the enormous resources that go into research and development for example, should that be to develop some medication that progress in medical knowledge would render useless in a couple of years, even if it had gone into the market? With the U.S, health spending billed to double over the next decade to over 4 trillion dollars per year, 20 cents/dollar spent on healthcare by 2016, 19.6 per cent of GDP, and according to 2006 estimates, current health spending 2.1 trillion dollars per year, or 16 cents in every dollar, concern about health expenditures are unlikely to wither[6]. Although attributable to population aging, at in least in part, as baby boomers become eligible for Medicare, spending growth on prescription drugs would also accelerate billed to increase an average of 8.6% yearly, or almost $500 billion in 2016, over twice current, 2006, figures[6]. According to the report, this increase in prescription drugs expenditure would be due to novel uses for older drugs, use of generics reaching a plateau, spending on new drugs meanwhile on the rise especially on diseases such as diabetes, and of heart diseases, and of other cardiovascular, and central nervous system diseases. Concerns regarding health spending would therefore target the pharmaceutical industry, among others, something the industry would have to be aware of and be able to handle the hostility that would emerge in certain quarters toward the industry. This underscores the point made earlier about image makeover, which as it becomes established would in no small measure help defray the costs accruable from such hostility. It also highlights the point made about benchmarking earlier. The pharmaceutical industry should therefore also be able to handle the changes that the potential increasing shift in the direction of the country's health system financing farther from employer-based to government based initiatives, Medicare's growth for example, faster than private insurance, would wrench on the industry vis-à-vis the ease or otherwise of paying for escalating healthcare costs. This could create added pressure on the industry regarding some blaming it for the funding woes, which even that the current 26.4% of the country's healthcare cost the individual pays would be less, 25% by 2016, and Medicare Part D reduces the prescription drugs burden, would unlikely change, as out of pocket expenses for those on private insurance would increase. With these out of pocket expenses including those on drugs, and spending on hospital and physician care also likely to increase, pharmaceutical firms would therefore likely continue to be the culprit to a large extent, for the health spending problems that would be evident in many different health services domains.

Interestingly, the report also noted that Americans would be keen to pay the

high price for current and new healthcare information and communication technologies, which is a crucial point that the pharmaceutical industry should factor into its strategizing. As we noted earlier, there is convergence to a more or less extent of the interests of the stakeholders in the healthcare delivery process, the role that these technologies would lay in which would be significant, evident in the findings in the study regarding the willingness of Americans to pay for technology applied to healthcare delivery, mentioned above. The increasingly widespread diffusion of healthcare information and communication technologies (ICT) would have far-reaching consequences for the pharmaceutical industry that it needs to be cognizant of well in advance. This is because these technologies would profoundly influence healthcare delivery, at the preventive, curative, and rehabilitative levels, new policy formulations and implementation resulting from which would cut across not just the health, but the pharmaceutical, insurance, and other industries related to the healthcare delivery enterprise. It is also instructive that there are over 300 medicines currently in development to treat or prevent a variety of rare diseases, as a new report that the Pharmaceutical Research and Manufacturers of America (PhRMA), recently released showed [7]. It is also pertinent that the Pharmaceutical Research and Manufacturers of America (PhRMA) represents key pharmaceutical research and biotechnology companies in the U.S, these firms investing an estimated $43 billion in 2006 in discovering and developing new drugs, industry wide research, and spending in the same year up to $55.2 billion. The National Institutes of Health projects about 6,000 rare diseases, one that affects less than 200,000 people, with 25 million individuals affected in the U.S. There is no doubt about the commitment of the pharmaceutical industry to the convergence mentioned earlier considering this report, and that prior to now, rare diseases have had non-existent or limited treatment options, progress inching along, over 160 medicines for their treatment approved since 1995, versus 108 ten years before, and just, ten years before then[7]. With 303 medicines now in human clinical trials or expecting approval by the FDA, it is doubtless that we should only chastise the pharmaceutical industry, considering the ethico-moral background of its efforts in this regard, not to mention its substantial research and development (R&D) and other investments. The patients with these conditions, and their families would doubtless recognize the efforts resulting in the development of a monoclonal antibody for chronic sarcoidosis, an immune system disorder, or for gene therapy for cystic fibrosis, or for the treatment of Lennox-Gastaut syndrome, severe epilepsy, and so should the rest of us. A point that Sharon F. Terry, MA, president, and CEO of the Genetic Alliance, which co-released the report, made eloquently. She says, "The companies undertaking the difficult and costly effort of developing drugs for rare disorders are making a profound impact on the lives of individuals and families with rare disorders...They focus on the question 'what matters' for people living every day with these diseases." Diane Edquist Dorman, vice president for public policy at the National Organization for Rare Disorders (NORD), which also co-released the study says, "NORD thanks the pharmaceutical industry for all it has accomplished over the past quarter century, and we look forward to working with PhRMA to address the challenges to be faced in the next 25 years." The significance of the Orphan Drug Act of 1983, which offer tax relief and some market exclusivity for firms developing an orphan drug also deserves mention, with the increased drug approvals for rare diseases since 1983 it spawned, 1,679 designated orphan drugs, although not all approved as of January 10, 2007. Indeed, the numbers of orphan drugs would likely increase with increasing knowledge of the genome, and emergence of potent novel technologies. That the pharmaceutical industry must continue to work towards playing its part in the 'comity' crucial to the progress of society and of humankind as our efforts to assure the delivery of qualitative health services evolve over time as it simultaneously faces the challenges within the industry and external to it that in some cases threaten its very survival. In the U.S., for example, intense lobbying is underway in Congress by the agents of the U.S. generic pharmaceutical industry, who want a patent law provision that they allege unfairly favors brand-name drug firms, expunged s. The law in the U.S., gives half a year market exclusivity to the first generic pharmaceutical firm that succeeds in challenging a brand-name patent, although the brand-name firm with the original patent could launch its 'authorized generic' versions during this period via third parties or subsidiaries. Sales of these authorized generics could undermine those of authorized generics substantially, the generic drug manufacturer's loss in profits during the exclusivity period sometimes over 60%, which explains the intense lobbying activities that aim to stop the marketing/selling of the authorized generics. Whether as some say these lobbyists should rather focus on President Bush's recent proposal requiring generic drug makers to pay user fees to FDA as they contend the lobby would fail in Congress is another matter, as is the contention that authorized generics foster competition, and they reduce prices, making drugs more affordable, hence more accessible to many. This yet others claim use fees would unlikely do, with authorized generics lurking. These and many other issues would remain contentious in the pharmaceutical industry and would require resolution by the industry, to leave room for attention to other equally important issues that in fact bother on the very existence of the industry. Thus, it inability to catch up with the fundamental evolutionary changes in the health sector that could profoundly influence the core of healthcare delivery itself, could potentially be sufficiently disruptive for the pharmaceutical industry to be threatening. At the end of the day, the industry would still have to contend with the most existentialist of all the issues it faces, that of its continued relevance in an ever-changing healthcare delivery milieu. The more successfully it does the likelier would it not just guarantee its survival, but also influence healthcare delivery enough to be a key player in the direction the latter moves. In other words, the pharmaceutical industry would need to continue to revalidate itself against in its strategic intent to remain needed, for healthcare delivery itself to survive.

References

1. Timmermans K (2007) Monopolizing clinical trial data: Implications and trends. *PLoS Med* 4(2):e02.

2. Available at: http://www.usatoday.com/money/industries/health/2007-02-14-fda-generics-usat_x.htm
Accessed on March 3, 2007

3. Available at:

http://www.medicalnewstoday.com/medicalnews.php?newsid=63194
Accessed on March 3, 2007

4. Available at: http://www.iom.edu/?id=37339 Accessed on March 3, 2007

5. Available at: http://www.usatoday.com/money/industries/health/drugs/2007-02-14-fda-budget-usat_x.htm Accessed on March 3, 2007

6. Poisal JA, Truffer C, Smith S, Sisko A, Cowan A, Keehan S, Dickensheets B. Health Spending Projections Through 2016: Modest Changes Obscure Part D's Impact. *Health Affairs*, doi: 10.1377/hlthaff.26.2.w242 (Published online February 21, 2007)

7. Available at: http://www.phrma.org/rarediseases/ Accessed on March 4, 2007

8. Available at:

http://www.northjersey.com/page.php?qstr=eXJpcnk3ZjczN2Y3dnFlZUVFeXk2
MTAmZmdiZWw3Zjd2cWVlRUV5eTcwODQ2MTkmeXJpcnk3ZjcxN2Y3dnFlZ
UVFeXky Accessed on March 4, 2007

What Does Health Matter?

Progress made in reforming labor and product markets has led to reduced

unemployment in Europe. Economic growth in many of the most developed countries in the world is impressive, but easing up on reforms could compromise long-term growth, according to the Organization for Economic Cooperation and Development (OECD). In the preface to the latest edition of its annual *Going for Growth* report, the organization's Chief Economist, Jean-Philippe Cotis, warned against cyclical buoyancy in continental Europe and Asian OECD countries siring complacency, urging Governments to continue with reforms that would increase productivity and job creation₁. There is no doubt that eschewing hindrance to labor force partaking and job creation would augment living standards, which opening up product and financial markets to increased competition would enhance, not to mention the shift it would spawn of the national income into increased wages and job formation from the corporate bottom line. The recommendations along these lines by the OECD were more specifically for continental Europe, the emphasis more on increasing productivity and on product-markets' liberalization, in particular network industries and in services, for lower-income countries, and for Japan and Switzerland. The report applauded the performance of the labor markets in English-speaking countries in general but noted that they need to improve skill levels, particularly via improvements in secondary education, and that many European Union (EU) countries need to brace higher-education systems to improve graduation rates and, in certain instances, even research and teaching quality. These recommendations raise critical issues for example the effect on the health of individuals and on a country's overall health status as judged by important health indicators such as disease prevalence, infant mortality rates, and life expectancy, and the effects of these direct, and indirect, on its economy. Would there be differential health implications of opening up the labor markets, for example, and what could this portend for healthcare costs and for health spending, and would it necessitate any, perhaps significant changes in health policy? With some convinced, that unchecked immigration is the main obstacle to economic growth in their countries, what are the prospects of the continuity of reforms in such countries essential to their sustained economic progress? What would be the challenges to employer-sponsored health insurance and indeed, to health services provision for the potentially teeming immigrants and what would be the implications for the entire economy of shifts in access to health services resultant? What political and economic barriers could be holding back structural reforms given these and other circumstances peculiar to certain jurisdictions and what measures would need taken to overcome them, hence promote and implement reforms? With it being clear, that ongoing differences in employment rates between countries, account in the main, for the experiential gaps in GDP per capita, evident also of the variance in the underpinnings of their policy and institutional frameworks, that we should explore the mechanics of this variance on employment outcomes is no doubt crucial in assuring reform continuity. It is thus, necessary to understand the interplay of factors on which the emergent labor and employment indicators depend, and via which their cross-interplay with other factors, for example, in the health domain, also significantly influence these and other salient economic indicators. This would reveal, among others, how each jurisdiction could employ knowledge of this interplay of indicators for examples of labor costs and taxation, health expenditure, labor and product market regulation, and for unemployment, disability, and illness support, in appropriate policy formulation and implementation. Jurisdictions would be able to couple for example the importance of easing or eliminating competition-limiting regulations in product markets, with that of fostering knowledge and skills acquisition, the latter that annuls the slowing of innovation diffusion of the former, negating of which also the consequent reduction in information and communications technologies investments, and in inward foreign direct investment. The potential for jeopardizing the achievement of the dual healthcare delivery objectives (DHDO) of qualitative health services provision, cost-effectively and efficiently, and indeed, spelt out more vividly, without increasing and in fact reducing healthcare costs, hence health spending, also evident considering the significant role these technologies play in so doing for example. The potential benefits of product market deregulation in driving productivity and economic prosperity would thus become increasingly clearer, as would their potential effect on health services provision, and by extension on the health of individuals and the country's overall health, in material and human terms. We would begin to appreciate in full the dynamics of the healthcare delivery/healthcare information and communications dyadic, and the centrality of the healthcare consumer in the symbiosis it represents, whose implications for market forces operations are crucial to the interplay of indicators mentioned above, differences in which are crucial to employment outcomes, and essentially, a country's wealth. The importance of knowledge and skills' acquisition as a cross-sectoral attribute would also become clearer as the tendency, of this centrality to influence the dyadic either way depends crucially on this attribute, in particular regarding rectifying the characteristically pervasive information asymmetry in the health sector. In tandem with the generativist tendency to innovative technologies of such acquisition, would emerge the true potential of this symbiotic dyadic to drive health services provision positively. The interplay of persistent paradigmatic shifts in the clinical domain that knowledge engenders stimulate innovative technological solutions among others, to novel challenges occasioned by enduring change, catalytic to a bi-directional augmentation of the elements of either component of the dyadic. In what more apposite milieu could these mechanisms play out than one competitive? Would it therefore be unreasonable to adduce the potential harm to not just health services provision, but to the economy to handle successfully the unemployment vicissitudes, in other words, to compromise the economy overall, not creating the enabling policies and institutional settings for competition not just to survive, but also to thrive?

I t is imperative under the prevailing circumstances to start to conceptualize

healthcare delivery in its full ramifications. For so long we have paid literally lip service to the importance of health in our affairs, but we seem to be in a bind, subjugating what we inherently recognize as crucial. Part of the problem is linguistic, the epitaph of health subsumed under an amorphous social services plaque on an obscure tombstone some would argue, the resource-guzzler connotation, a veritable traffic diversion even in a surreal mystic playground in an arroyo ordinarily traversed incognito. With such venom for its ilk, is it any wonder we would rather dodge, than confront it? On the other hand, are we burnt-out trying? The U.S' health spending projected in 2006 at \$2.1 trillion, 16% of its gross domestic product (GDP), projected to double over the next decade from current levels to reach \$4.1 trillion, which would be about twenty cents of every dollar spent, certainly does not seem trivial[2]. Not even that the economists/actuaries from the Office of the Actuary at the Centers for Medicare and Medicaid Services (CMS) in their annual forecasting report, also forecast the average annual health spending growth would remain steady at 6.9% between 2006 and 2016, even, fall from 6.9% in 2005 to 6.8% in 2006, the fourth consecutive spending-lull year, trivializes it. In the end, which might explain the debate in Congress of a Bush administration proposal to cut \$26 billion from Medicaid spending over the next five years, we would still agonize over the country's health spending. Yet, a recent research emphasized the need rather to focus on fundamental programs reform to expunge interstate variations in benefits and support the states in managing soaring health costs[3]. Recently also, researchers have shown that the projected fall in employer-sponsored insurance, and seniors' long-term care needs regardless, average Medicaid spending as a share of national health spending would be 16.6% between 2006 and 2025, same, 16.5% as in 2005, then rise slowly to 19.0% by 2045[4], increases estimated government revenue growth would be sufficient to sustain. What we glean from these studies then, essentially the likelihood of health services provision to the deprived, and indeed, to all, if it took the required measures to slash costs where they really should be, speaks volume, literally. It brings to the fore the point made earlier regarding the need to achieve the dual healthcare delivery objectives, and the important role that healthcare ICT would play in so doing, not to mention the resulting positive effect on the healthcare delivery/healthcare information and communications technologies dyadic. Thus, if we concurred with these observations and took the necessary measures, we would be highlighting the importance of health not only in our lives, but also in the economic progress or otherwise of our country. Is it not apt for example to establish appropriate policies for healthcare ICT diffusion, which that whose benefits realized in full might have up to a ten-year lag based on the experiences of other industries that have implemented information technologies pervasively, could be a costly delay not so doing in earnest, is instructive? Besides not intuitive, why would we want to tarry on an issue that compromises our economy as we do, if we were not to discountenance the implications for productivity of an unhealthy workforce, and the perpetuation of the very businesses whose operations pivot the economy? How would such businesses be competitive at home, not to mention in the global marketplace, if they were unproductive, or were only so at enormous costs, which made them essentially unprofitable? How could we inculcate in our youths for example, the basics of these crucial epiphenomena, on whose lucid articulation the full appreciation of the complex interplay of health in our economy by not just youths, but also all else depends? Does this not speak to the differential modality of the expression of this complexity whose very essence the point about the widespread diffusion of information technologies, in an age the social web, reigns, for example? It is thus not just exigent, but indeed, imperative that we explore in our efforts to highlight the significance of health, contextual information dissemination portals considering that we conceptualize knowledge and skills acquisition in essentially generic-on-specific terms. This again, stresses the need for an equally broad based framework for policy formulation aimed at reinforcing competition in products/service markets, in achieving our goals of further reducing unemployment and improving productivity, both incumbent on collateral initiatives to improve healthcare delivery in access and quality terms, among others, as herein discussed. This underscores the contention over the role and extent of government involvement in reinforcing competition, the role, again, in the health sector, that healthcare information and communications technologies could play in this regard evident. In other words, we need to recognize the limits of regulations, and as the OECD report mentioned above noted, enforcing competition laws varies among member states, these laws still obstacles to competition in many economic sectors, in particular the services sector, and in network industries not necessarily facilitative of access to networks, and even discourage capacity expansion. Whereas, and in keeping with our conceptualization of the centrality of the healthcare consumer, market forces operational at different levels would promote competitiveness among healthcare providers for example, including in the use of these technologies to market distinctive value propositions that confer competitive edge. In this context, the question of which and to what extent government versus professional bodies regulate these activities becomes moot. Such an approach to regulation as opposed to wholesale government involvement in free-market market activities coincide with the core of the recommendations made by the OECD referred to above. Indeed, OECD, in the same report acknowledged that governments in many member states have established product/labor markets structural reforms intended to promote competition and productivity, some successfully, others thwarted by political fiat. It thus stressed the need for a thorough design and appraisal of the reform process, which underscores the potential for minimal government intervention being sine qua non for these reforms to work, exemplified by the healthcare delivery/healthcare ICT symbiotic dyadic with elements that essentially feed on each other to create ongoing, albeit incremental process improvement in both. This is in contradistinction to the observation made in the OECD report regarding the network industries earlier mentioned. This is not to trivialize the political in the reform process, evident in the opposition by Governors, in the US at their meeting on February 25, 2007, to President Bush's budget for a health care program, which aims to insure millions of children of working poor families, stressing their concern over budget shortfalls further swelling the ranks of the uninsured 5. That the Governors want guarantees of funding, an estimated $745 million for State Children's Health Insurance Program (SCHIP), which covers 6 million people, mostly children, but which in some states now includes adults in these families, over half a million, with funds running out in Georgia for example, in March, prior to the new budget in October, is understandable. This is besides the contention that Bush's program would shortchange SCHIP by $10 billion to $15 billion over the next five years, which among others would jeopardize state efforts to initiate universal health care programs, insuring all children, the starting point of which for most states. With the Bush administration, emphasizing not just that SCHIP should focus on underprivileged children, and not all children, but also that it should exclude adults, and that in fact, states with surpluses sharing funds with those with deficits would eliminate the short-term shortfalls it is not difficult to see the likely protracted nature of the looming controversy. This controversy also buttresses the point about exploring the interplays mentioned earlier, with for example, the importance of coverage for children, within the framework of a vision of a potentially healthier future populace, and of that of the prospects, even now, of the intra-family health and wellness cascade that such a populace of children would spawn. In other words, we could be staving off healthcare costs, hence spending down the road, which the exhausted mother or care-giver for example, would incur nurturing a perpetually ill child, not to mention two, perhaps even more, the potential to pull such caregivers down the economic ladder, laid off due to repeated absenteeism for example, real. Granted the complexities of working out a perfect arrangement for healthcare financing, every jurisdiction needs to devise these arrangements bearing in mind the interplay of factors with potential roller-coater effects on other aspects of the economy. This accentuates the significance of the continual exploration mentioned earlier of these factors, and the need to augment each at its particular level as part of the overall efforts to improve the whole, and meet the generic objectives that we set out to achieve. This ongoing exploratory process predicate on the assumption, which we must also make that no health system could ever be perfect, and that the best we could do would be to make ours as near-perfect as possible. That health systems or any system for that matter could never be perfect, itself is inherent in the nature of health systems, which must of necessity change, for example, due to new medical knowledge warranting a change in an established surgical procedure. These changes render current systems obsolete in a general sense, therefore, and make new ones to meet the challenges so created, necessary to implement.

It is this appreciation of the importance of change in our affairs that would

heighten that of the role of health in them also. It would help in situating the age-old contention over the role of government in free market economies, for example, wherein, the perfect scenario, with no taxes, no government interventions such as price fixing, license quotas and industry subsidies, in the context of health as a major driver of the economy. It would dismantle customary conceptualizations of health as a quarternary, or in some quarters, 'quinary' in primary, as we see the centrality of its role in the success of the industries in the traditional classificatory scheme. The announcement by the U.S Congress' Joint Committee on Taxation on March 01, 2007, that President Bush's health insurance proposals would cost taxpayers $526 billion through 2017, which some deem a form of tax increases, exemplifies these points, given the potential effects of such increases on individuals' disposable incomes, and on economic activities in the country in general[6]. Further, the plan essentially means treating the cost of an insurance policy, both employer's and the employee's payments, as taxable income, the result, workers' taxable wages sky bound. However, the president advocates a standard tax deduction for persons that purchase health insurance, those keeping policy costs less the new deduction receiving a tax break. Many believe that the current tax break for healthcare promotes more spending and that the tax-free benefit encourages people to buy the most inclusive policies offered, whereas the new tax change effective in FY2009, would slow health costs as individuals seek less costly insurance in order to receive a tax cut, which equally applies to employer-sponsored or self-purchased insurance. These developments are instructive in the context of the press release released the same day that personal income increased $108.1 billion, or 1.0 percent, and disposable personal income (DPI), personal income less personal current taxes, increased

$73.0 billion, or 0.8 percent, in January, versus an increase of $46.0 billion, or 0.5

percent, in December, by the Bureau of Economic Analysis[7]. Yet, according to the

press release, personal outlays such as personal consumption expenditures

(PCE), personal interest payments, and personal current transfer payments

increased $55.3 billion in January, versus an increase of $70.4 billion in

December. Additionally, personal saving, DPI less personal outlays, was a

negative $116.4 billion in January, versus a negative $134.2 billion in December,

and personal saving as a percentage of disposable personal income was a

negative 1.2 percent in January, versus a negative 1.4 percent in December.

Indeed, personal income increased 6.3 percent in 2006, from the 2005 to the 2006

annual level, versus an increase of 5.2 percent in 2005. DPI increased 5.4 percent,

versus an increase of 4.1 percent, PCE by 6.0 percent, versus an increase of 6.5

percent. Thus, on the one hand, developments such as bonus payments and stock

options gains enhanced private wage and salaries, those of government, pay rises

for federal civilian and military staff. On the other, negative personal saving

indicates personal outlays over and above disposable personal income, which

would likely be worse the less the personal income in the first place. What likely

effect would this have on individuals' ability to purchase health insurance vis-à-

vis the federal government's proposed tax cut for persons seeking less costly

insurance? As we noted earlier, should governments not be encouraging more

widespread healthcare coverage? These issues again highlight that of the nature

and extent of government intervention in free market operations mentioned

earlier. Considering the importance of pervasive healthcare coverage for the

economy, some would argue for significant government input regarding

regulations and related exercises to ensure the achievement of this goal, which

achievement is no doubt, crucial, but that government should intervene significantly others would contend. Indeed, some would advocate the intervention to be even across borders, pressure on China for example, whose increasingly pivotal role in the world economy they would consider necessary under certain circumstances to prevent adverse consequences on the global economy that could affect the country, directly or otherwise, exerting the pressure. Some would say for example that the increase in China's trade surplus by 67% in January 2007 would likely trigger such concerns. This is in particular regarding its low (undervalued) currency, the Yuan, many hold accountable, as it makes Chinese exports cheaper, in the main for it for example, as it did in January 2007, exporting $15.9bn (£8.2bn) more goods and services than it imported, versus $9.5bn for the same month in 2006[8]. Indeed, on February 09, 2007, the G7 finance minister from the world's foremost industrial countries urged China to make its currency more flexible. With China's, trade surplus with the European Union (EU) reaching $26.4bn in January 2007, that with the US, $23.41bn, and its overall trade surplus for 2006, $177.47bn, up 74% on 2005, su ch concerns could only increase. Is it therefore the case that government intervention in the free market, including in the operations of the healthcare delivery enterprise, is inevitable? Is this why in fact some would insist that the free market concept is a myth? In addition to such situations as mentioned above, that a recent New York Times/CBS News poll released on March 02, 2007, showed that most Americans want the federal government to guarantee health insurance to every American, in particular children, and are willing to pay higher taxes if necessary for this to happen, make these questions moot[9]. It is also instructive that this poll showed that access to affordable healthcare is topmost public domestic agenda, considered far more important than immigration, tax cuts, or traditional values promotion. Indeed, Americans were willing to make sacrifices to guarantee health insurance for all, such as paying up to $500 more in taxes per year. They even would jettison future tax cuts. Yet, the old division over universal health insurance persists, some would contend, in the main along the Republican/Democratic line, although in California, Gov. Arnold Schwarzenegger, who has proposed something akin to universal health coverage, is a Republican. Former Senator John Edwards is a Democratic presidential candidate and has proposed a compromise plan, which would require all to have insurance and employers to provide it or contribute to a fund that would. It is also instructive that although Democrats customarily support health coverage expansion, significant numbers of Republicans and independents also do according to this poll. This speaks to the fact that the public in fact increasingly believes that health indeed, matters, and with almost 47 million individuals in the country, or over 15% of its peoples lacking health insurance, an increase of 6.8 million from the 2000 figures, this is hardly surprising. The reason it is not is essentially rooted in the fundamental fact regarding humankind of the right to life, the tendency of the majority of peoples to want to live rather than to die, and this applies to persons worldwide. The significance of this fact for the questions we raised earlier concerning the nature and extent of government intervention in healthcare d elivery is profound. So is it for the future of health and healthcare delivery, not just in the U.S., but also in other countries around the world. We did mention earlier also that government intervention vis-à-vis those of key operators in the healthcare delivery enterprise would emerge. This emergence is partly the product of the operations of a variety of factors that counteract any tendency toward humankind being moribund. The zeal behind the findings of the poll mentioned above is also one capable of driving other actions of the healthcare consumer that would improve health services delivery in time. Such drivers would for example make the role of government in the potential catalytic bent of the widespread diffusion of healthcare information and communication technologies (ICT) in improving healthcare deliver, essentially facilitator-based. In other words, hardly would it be necessary for government to legislate, for example, the pervasive employment of healthcare ICT in the healthcare delivery enterprise, when the healthcare consumer would increasingly lean towards service providers that are, in effect ICT-enabled. This would be a differentiator of the increasingly sophisticated value propositions these providers, would have to offer to an equally more discerning clientele. Competition, therefore, would impel innovation, and improve healthcare delivery. The American public would therefore not have to experience such frustration by the state of affairs with their health services as to have to offer to pay even more taxes to fund and improve them. Who would blame them for example for overwhelmingly, as the poll showed, not just supporting the Children's Health Insurance Program, devised for low- and moderate-income children, which Congress has to renew this year, but also expanding it to cover all uninsured children, estimated currently at over eight million? Are they wrong to think, again indicated in the poll, that the lack of health insurance for many children was a "very serious" problem for the US? Are the responses not indicative of the subtle convergence of underlying forces, including those economic that assure the right to life mentioned earlier? The point here therefore, is that rather than agonize over the nature and role of government, we should enable the expression of this right by promoting the accentuation of the relevant forces cryptic or otherwise, crucial in so doing.

There is no doubt that it is troubling that, as the poll mentioned above showed, 25% of Americans with insurance indicated that someone in their household forfeited a medical test or treatment due to lack of insurance coverage, or that 60% of those without that someone in their household had, due to costs. Perhaps this explains why almost two thirds of those polled supported government guaranteeing health insurance, and many more that the country's health care system required deep-seated change or total shake-up, as it seems, blending both government and private involvement. Considering historical antecedents, the need for such a common ground is doubtless crucial in the country, the realization of which however, needs spelling out does not necessarily follow such dichotomous conceptualizations. This last point is significant here as it embodies the contents of the next stage in our efforts at highlighting the crucial role of health in our affairs, having established the first that it counts. If we concurred also that, the tendency is toward the right to life than otherwise, we would start to move closer to the realization of this second stage as well. In other words, and as applies to all other countries, chief among what holds progress back in healthcare delivery is our rigmarole on the subject itself. We expend precious time drawing arbitrary lines which if only we stepped back to tease out the fundamentals of the healthcare delivery enterprise, we would not only find absolutely disingenuous, but also that doing otherwise is absolutely harmless. It would be clear to us that we could without splitting hairs literally, on the mode of financing our health systems, not compromise the interests of stakeholders, in whatever domain, interests that often take center stage when the centrality of the healthcare consumer should, and to which latter we essentially bramble in acquiescing. Would it not be nice for more Americans to know the extent of private healthcare insurance in Canada, or for more Canadians to know that of government spending relative to private health insurance in the US? Even now, therefore, both these countries have a mix of public and private health insurance with a preponderance of one or the other although the perception of their health funding differs in the main, Canada, perceived as publicly funded, and the U.S., as privately-funded exclusively by many. The situation is the same in the UK, where there is increasing private-sector involvement in the country's National Health Service (NHS), perceived essentially by many as a publicly funded health system, and it is with other health systems worldwide. It is evident, however, that these distinctions would fade away over time, as the reality of the contemporary health system sets in, albeit with a little help from efforts such as advocated here, aimed at appreciating more fully, the essential elements of healthcare delivery within a perpetually changing operational milieu. This would be even more so as the milieu would one in which the operators would increasingly become discerning in their choices of services expected and rendered. Thus, a necessary next step having established the importance of health in our affairs would be that of ensuring the provision of qualitative and accessible services, without shearing the budget. This has nothing to do with the funding system of that health system, generically. In other words, every health system would have to strive to achieve these dual healthcare delivery objectives, to ensure that it meets the requirements for moving the motion forward of not just the health system, but also the entirety of our systems toward the realization of the right to exist. Each health jurisdiction has to focus on creating the enabling environment for the centrality of the healthcare consumer to take hold, which must predicate on empowering the healthcare consumer to make the correct choices regarding health issues. This would ensure the proper workings of supply and demand premises crucial to the emergence of the competitive environment, in turn necessary for the forward motion of the health system mentioned earlier. As we promote this competitiveness therefore, we simultaneously facilitate free market operations, making the need for government intervention minimal. In other words, the direction of the funding of our health systems would emerge in particular jurisdictions from the cumulative interplay of market forces operational. Considering the differences in these cumulative forces and the evolutionary pace of different jurisdictions, not to mention the prevailing circumstances in the health and related domains and in the non-health domains that nonetheless potentially affect healthcare delivery, we cannot overemphasize the significance of local flavor. Thus, the nature and extent of government involvement would depend on the peculiarities of jurisdictions that reflect the accumulation of institutions and infrastructures required to facilitate the complex transactions involved in the healthcare delivery enterprise, including their interplay with the ongoing requirements that current circumstances dictate. These local considerations though would need to be within the broad framework applicable at the generic level to for example, all jurisdictions within a country, and as determined in some cases by the circumstances prevalent even outside its borders. The basic requirement and indeed, starting point of placing the healthcare consumer at the center of the healthcare delivery universe so to speak, which implies the freedom to choose regarding health services provision, and other matters, becomes imperative in making the others work. Implicit in this empowerment of the healthcare consumer is the inculcation of knowledge and skills essential to such decision-making, one that would be rational and relevant to the realization of the overall goals of the health system in the particular jurisdiction. This makes the inculcation of such knowledge in the best interest of not just the healthcare consumer but also the health system, which underscores the point we made earlier about serving the interests of all healthcare stakeholders without necessarily heightening the intensity of government regulation and hegemony over the health system. It is no doubt not, what we want that about a million persons await admissions to NHS facilities and 800,000 are waiting for medical procedures in Canada currently[10]. Nor do we want to see governments spending increasing amounts of their gross domestic product (GDP) on healthcare delivery as happening in many countries, particularly in the developed world lately. Thus, we want to ensure access to care, cost-effectively and efficiently. Bearing the advice of the OECD in mind, we would have to factor in the equation access to care by the immigrant workers that would swell our workforce too. Our approach to health insurance, whether public or private would need to consider such issues, and as we noted earlier, would vary by jurisdictional peculiarities. What would our health system benefit from an increasing number of unhealthy intended-workers, who could not just access curative, but also preventive services, not to mention our economic system? Yet, it makes a lot of difference that they are now within our borders with their health problems potentially a drain on our resources as we would have to foot the bulk of the bill in the end anyway, when they have become even more ill, brought on a stretcher to our hospital emergency rooms. The point here is to emphasize the third stage of the significance of the potential economic issues that belie the presumed healthcare delivery cameo. In other words, as we let immigrant workers into the country, to help build and fortify our economy, we acquire responsibilities beyond paying the wages, including health services provision, among others. Put differently, an important aspect of cross-border immigration critical to the progress of contemporary economies is healthcare delivery, and each health jurisdiction, in consonance with the other domains in the overall jurisdiction would have to be cognizant of this fact, and take the necessary measures to accommodate the newcomers in their policy formulation and service planning efforts. We should at various management levels both in the health sector, and in related sectors, therefore, consider these issues as essential components of the requirements to achieve the dual healthcare delivery objectives (DHDO), in the process of working towards actualizing the contributions to our overall economy, of the healthcare delivery enterprise. In other words, we should start to view health as not just 'business as usual' but within the context of the very survival of our economy and our country. Health would then begin to matter to us in a very different way, one which does not constrain us, but opens vistas hitherto constrained, yet that would revolutionize the way we not just deliver health but indeed, other services to our peoples.

The point is that of a comprehensive outlook to health becoming a required

mindset among not just policy makers but all healthcare stakeholders in healthcare delivery now and in future. That hospitals have a legal requirement to provide healthcare an individual's ability to pay, nonetheless, and that doctors, and other healthcare professionals, even if not legally so bound, are ethically, and morally bound to provide such services too, is instructive vis-à-vis our desire to provide qualitatively and affordable health services for immigrants and citizens alike. We ought therefore to start thinking seriously about reducing the tax burden occasioned on those with health insurance and in general the taxpayer, everyone including the immigrant worker not having health insurance coverage, the costs of such uncompensated care in the US for example up to 5% of the country's overall health expenditure[11]. This is not to mention the counter-productiveness regarding our goals of boosting our workforce with young and healthy persons, including from abroad, with these same persons, typically likely to discount health insurance. This is also not to mention the resulting additional increase in healthcare costs, hence spending that the adverse selection the actions of these young persons cause, with insurance premiums skyrocketing, the old and infirm mainly buying health insurance. Thus ensuring that we create the enabling environment for widespread healthcare coverage is in the interests of all, and in the long term, assists in the achievement of our dual healthcare delivery objectives on the one hand, and of that to secure the contributions of the health sector to the overall economic progress of our country on the other. It is not always clear the intricacies of the relationships between health and the economy, yet, this relationship should be one we all should know about and appreciate. This could, by revealing to us, even as individuals, the role we could play, via as simple measures as living healthier lives, and seeking prompt and effective treatment for our health conditions, in buoying the economy of our country, inculcate in us a sense of ownership. The sense would not just be of our health and us but also of the affairs of our country, the effects that could be quite profound. Indeed, part of our efforts in this regard should commence from as early as possible in life, the endowments imbibed by the youths with potentially longer lasting effects than started later in life, although this is not to say that we could not start at any point in the life cycle. In fact, we should start right away to promote the appreciation of the value of health among the citizenry in novel ways, strategizing based on assumptions rooted in the fundamentals we have touched upon in our discussion here, among others, for example. Our efforts to place the healthcare consumer at the center of the scheme of things in healthcare delivery would therefore, and as earlier noted predicate on the free-flow of information among all healthcare stakeholders. This would among others, focus on all aspects of health and healthcare delivery, in particular emphasizing those that under-discussed but are in fact crucial to the success of our healthcare delivery endeavors. There are indeed, other important issues that would confront each health jurisdiction, outside the generic for example in the US whether to expand or constrict subsidies, the former many state legislatures embrace, essentially as it helps maximize federal funds receipt, fostering cross-state costs deferment, as opposed to the single-payer health system as in Canada, for example. Yet, subsidies could crowd-out unsubsidized coverage, discouraging employer-sponsored coverage, which is why some would context the idea of expanding Medicaid up the earnings ladder, for example, or without restrictions, the dependence potential on the program now by even more. Each health jurisdiction would have to confront its peculiar problems and devise the most appropriate solutions to them, within the general framework that we have here argued applies to all health systems. In lieu of government-run health systems for example, some states in the US, in a bid to offer universal coverage have instituted a variety of employer mandates essentially compelling businesses to fund health coverage for their employees or contribute to a special fund to do so. Besides being the subject of litigations in many of these states, the overall result is unlikely going to be favorable for the employees as employers would find ways to offset the healthcare costs. The result also would likely be unfavorable for the entire economy, as the measures, for examples layoffs, automation, even outsourcing, taken might, by extension also hurt the entire economy. Some states, such as Massachusetts, have individual mandates, over which the question of individual liberty looms large, not to mention potential expansion of mandated benefits courtesy of lobbyists, and enforceability, in particular among the underprivileged many that do not have health insurance and for whom such programs aim to offer coverage. We cannot overemphasize the significance of addressing these issues by different health jurisdictions, but perhaps more importantly of so doing considering the basics some of which we here discussed as the veritable wellsprings of the initiatives further up the epigenetic ladder towards achieving the dual healthcare delivery objectives that every health system should set out to achieve. Healthcare delivery in our time has become a complex endeavor that requires serious focus by all concerned, the earlier we pay attention to the critical issues increasingly proving to be strategic in achieving our goals as opposed to the later. The question is no longer, whether health matters, but how we could make it even more effective and efficient in contributing its quota to our lives and to the economic progress of our country.

References

1. Available at: http://www.oecd.org/growth/goingforgrowth2007 Accessed on
February 25, 2007

2. Poisal, JA, Truffer, C, Smith, S, Sisko, A, Cowan, C, Keehan, S, Dickensheets, B,
and National Health Expenditures Team, Health Spending Projections Through
2016: Modest Changes Obscure Part D's Impact, *Health Affairs* Web Exclusive,
February 21, 2007
Available at:

http://content.healthaffairs.org/cgi/content/abstract/hlthaff.26.2.w242 Accessed
on February 25, 2007

3. Holahan, J and Alan Weil. Toward Real Medicaid Reform [*Health Affairs* 26, no.
2 (2007): w254-w270 (published online 23 February 2007;
10.1377/hlthaff.26.2.w254)]
Available at:
http://content.healthaffairs.org/cgi/content/full/hlthaff.26.2.w254v1/DC1
Accessed on February 25, 2007

4. Kronick, R, and David Rousseau Is Medicaid Sustainable? Spending
Projections For The Program's Second Forty Years [*Health Affairs* 26, no. 2 (2007):
w271-w287 (published online 23 February 2007; 10.1377/hlthaff.26.2.w271)]

Available at:

http://content.healthaffairs.org/cgi/content/abstract/hlthaff.26.2.w271v1 Accessed on February 25, 2007

5. Available at: http://www.usatoday.com/news/washington/2007-02-26-governors-kids-health_x.htm Accessed on February 26, 2007.

6. Available at: http://www.sfgate.com/cgi-bin/article.cgi?file=/n/a/2007/02/28/national/w145630S19.DTL&type=printable Accessed on March 1, 2007

7. Available at: http://www.bea.gov/newsreleases/national/pi/pinewsrelease.htm Accessed on March 1, 2007

8. Available at: http://news.bbc.co.uk/go/pr/fr/-/2/hi/business/6353183.stm Accessed on March 1, 2007

9. Available at: http://www.nytimes.com/2007/03/02/washington/02poll.html?_r=2&adxnnl=1&oref=slogin&ref=todayspaper&adxnnlx=1172854800-P38Y6lVXPm2ZPHHiIj5W2g&pagewanted=print Accessed on March 02, 2007

10. Cannon M, Tanner, M. *Healthy Competition: What's Holding Back Health Care and How to Free It* (Washington: Cato Institute: 2005), pp. 36–37.

11. Greg Scandlen, "The Pitfalls of Mandating Health Insurance," *Council for Affordable Health Insurance's Issues & Answers*, no. 135 (April 2006).

A Mystic Health Voyage

An examination of the fundamental architectures of the human experience

would reveal an approach to constructing the political in which the contemporary generalizations evident in the operations of its players might situate. The social for example becomes distinct from the customary public versus private, even if the context vis-à-vis both remains fuzzy, and given the seeming cacophony, that mystifies both also the portended. The debates over the nature and extent of authority becomes moot, as the blurring of authority itself given the fuzziness of the elements of the situations purportedly to control perplexes more than edifies. That we could not jettison the exigencies ominous in this scenario is retiring, and we struggle to reconstruct the intellectual framework on which the architectures predicate, cognizant of the costs of delay tarrying. The existential rubrics that underpin much of the prevalent themes in every generic domain become evident, and the epigenesis contingent upon which, albeit even if cryptic is at once, also evident. As does the interchange characteristic of the expression, not to mention the evolution of each domain, our perception of the value inherent in the domains sires tendencies in us, which by default aggregate to illuminate the grandeur of the totality of this expression. We start to enjoy the knowledge and appreciation of the transactions between expressional modes contributory to this manifestation, in keeping with the emotional attributes required for the incremental expression of our existential goals. We discountenance other tendencies that result in moribund materializations, in disengaging to engage each action apposite to such aversions that we necessarily embrace qua motion in the direction of the appropriate manifestations. In effect, we establish the necessary structures and institutions within the appropriate framework to enable the realization of our goals, which for example in the health domain, we characteristically consider dual, given the prevalent health spending patterns, which would no doubt concern many, the delivery of qualitative health services cost-effectively, and efficiently. The elements of quality we would also characterize to embody the values of the health services that our peoples have come to expect, which we could safely assume, would be at the level of a need, which we could equally assume would be increasingly complex and sophisticated. We would have no qualms in so doing since the essential basis of the centrality of the healthcare consumer would be clear to us all given the efforts prior, efforts cognizant of the need to rectify the pervasive information asymmetry characteristic of the healthcare industry, for example, the atavistic relic of entrenched paternalism that the operators themselves struggle to eschew. We acquire a new mindset that impels us to address the asymmetry from an early age, even if we did not constrain our efforts to the kindergarten. We recognize the stupendous transactional costs constitutive substantially of the gross national product (GNP) in many developed countries yet rectifiable, so doing sine qua non to a generic approach to addressing the information asymmetry issue crucial to reducing significantly the costs of the transactions, considering the numbers, varieties, and complexities of which in the healthcare delivery enterprise, would be instructive. It would thus behoove us to formulate the appropriate policies to ensure the widespread diffusion for example of efficient and cost-effective means to accomplish this goal, knowing full well, the disparities in the resources our peoples could avail imbibing the information, knowledge and skills intended for inculcation. Our efforts would thus include contextualizing information symmetry promotion wherein the increasing preeminence of the social over the public and the private for example, would serve us well, as we employ the resources technological and otherwise that foster this trend. In other words, we would be better able to appreciate that the roots of the centrality of the healthcare consumer for example, would spawn an intellectual awareness cascade that would galvanize action indeed, beyond policy levels, to the investment for example in the relevant initiatives to operationalize these policies. The corollary therefore is true that we would likelier become so motorized situating policy within such fundamental frameworks of our existential experience that we seem to have for so long suppressed. The political would become more cogent as its elocutions become more meaningful, rooted in the realities of this existential experience, the veracity of actions in tandem with their sources in the acclamations we all make. Even rancor would no longer be un-understandable, itself the marshalling in deserved eloquence immediately evident of the richness of the goals sought. We would no longer see deferment in disagreement as stalling, but an opportunity for a refresher in which the issues would re-emerge in a novel form, with more credible content. That milieu would foster debates on issues that would reflect the interests that we would rather serve, than allow to rot, as we did, fiddle away, oblivious to the potential harm that lurks ahead. It would be obvious for example that we would be better able to achieve the dual healthcare delivery objectives (DHDO) mentioned earlier, not ignoring the facts, regarding the contributions say the widespread implementation and utilization of healthcare information and communication technologies (healthcare ICT) could make in so doing. This would make it unnecessary to compel all healthcare stakeholders to invest in these technologies, which now for example, is hardly the case, indeed, the paradoxical anxieties some feel so doing, exemplifies the potential of a reverse existential experience to the tendencies in the main inherent in our preferences. This might indeed, be a manifestation of the need to rectify the pervasive information asymmetry mentioned earlier, which itself highlights that to engage in the sort of exercise we here do, examining the basic architectures of the human experience. In a generic sense, therefore, we confront our lassitude in ensuring the full appreciation of the human experience in earnest, recognizing the delay we have already, not suited to the expediency that the realization of our goals demands. We become even more acutely aware of the benefits accruable from so doing, for example, which could ensure the continuing validity of some of our most cherished values, for example helping us tease out the nature and extent of government intervention in the processes that interplay to result in the goals we seek. It thus opens up debates on the elements of the nature of free-market as opposed to mixed economy, relevant to now, freeing us from outmoded dogmas for example in the economic domain. We start to see no contradiction in opening up our markets and expanding our labor force, increasing its sophistication, and our economic progress, but in fact see both being complementary. In the process, we become aware of the need to factor in addition to wages, health services provision, and social welfare for the teeming immigrants that arrive at our shores to buttress our economies. Ou r conceptualizations of issues become broader-based in keeping with our new realities. Therefore, we come more to terms with the true meaning of change and of its import for our journey toward realizing our goals. That we cannot avoid change is starker, although we accept it with sublimity, and this becomes the locus of the process-cycle analyses we commit to for example, in a decomposition/exposition cycle that we engage in fully cognizant that our health systems could never be perfect, the reason, at least in part, inherent in change. We are in effect able to accept and indeed, confront the challenges that our health systems present as they undergo the changes imposed from within and without the systems. It becomes clearer to us that at the fast pace of knowledge acquisition in the medical field, we cannot but expect disruptions, in the status quo, regarding healthcare delivery. This realization would demand the analyses of the processes to determine the mechanisms by which we could update them to meet the requirements imposed by change, hence make the health systems function cost-effectively and efficiently given these new requirements. It would therefore, be more acceptable for us, to invest in say healthcare ICT, required to facilitate the complicated transactions constitutive of healthcare delivery, and which would ensure that we continue to realize the dual healthcare delivery objectives that we set out to achieve. Our exploration would therefore open up the potential lurking in our systems, which we have hitherto perhaps even studiously ignored political expediencies no longer able to account for initiatives that the expectations of our health systems by the public would demand. Nor would the public have to offer solutions that reflect the workings of the fundamental underpinnings of the human experience such as the findings in a recent New York Times/CBS News poll[1], given alternatives that are more effective.

The poll showed that most Americans not only want the federal government

to guarantee health insurance to every American, especially children, but that they are willing to pay higher taxes, as much as $500 more in taxes per year and indeed to forfeit going future tax cuts, so to do. Not only are the adverse effects of higher taxes at the individual and national levels ominous, in economic and other terms, that we could achieve the desired goals implementing measures geared towards realizing the dual healthcare delivery objectives for example, could make higher taxation unnecessary. Nonetheless, the offer underscores the crucial point we have made here, namely that the tendency to the right to life that we share in the main, is a crucial conceptual starting point for exploring what we have thus far termed the existential in our construction of the architectures of the human experience. From this conceptual root would emerge an edifice that would form the backbone of our outlook to healthcare issues that we would have to deal with at jurisdictional levels, the local flavor of which, the sophistication of the edifice would inevitably be adequate to savor as solutions emerge within a solid framework. Indeed, this framework would be applicable generically say in the health domain to all jurisdictions. Thus, as we explore the issues germane to the motion of health services provision in the appropriate direction, which the fundamentals determine, specifically against that opposite to survival we revisit our infrastructures and institutions, to ensure they could meet the challenges imposed by change as earlier mentioned. In facilitating the utilization by the healthcare consumer in keeping with consolidating the centrality of the position of the healthcare consumer, it would become obvious that we need to ensure openness and accountability for the rational decision-making that the information acquired by the healthcare consumer engendered to be meaningful in practical terms. In other words, the healthcare consumer would therefore need to have an opportunity to exit the system as necessary, or have a voice in it in addition to system having a hierarchy system that ensures accountability as Paul (1992) observed[2]. We would, in the process be contributing toward enhancing the quality of the health systems, hence to our prospects of achieving the DHDO. The centrality of the healthcare consumer also makes it necessary for individual healthcare stakeholders to perform optimally, a tacit testimony to the underlying market forces that are operational. The operations of market forces as we noted earlier, being necessarily imperfect, some would contend explains the concept of the mixed economy, even if our goals should rather be to make it ever more perfect, which the exploration we are herewith engaged underscores. Thus, by backing our concept of the centrality of the healthcare consumer up with the appropriate actions, we would be contributing substantially toward making market operations increasingly closer to perfection in the health sector, with individual stakeholders as noted earlier, obliged to enhance value propositions to remain in the market. The healthcare consumer would not necessarily demand this, but it would be the rational end-result of the variety of processes, including a more discerning clientele, more affordable healthcare ICT, due to more pervasiveness, the results of promotional efforts, and paradigmatic shifts in healthcare delivery, in the healthcare delivery enterprise. Not even this is the final form, could one be emphatic postulating, but it is no doubt an important element of the process that leads towards it, if it in fact exists, considering the strategic objectives we pursue are fluid, depending on our circumstances, which might be dramatically different in a century, even as the right to life remains central. This places the onus on us to ensure in approaching change that we do not for lack of a full appreciation of its result, jeopardize our very status and the benefits to pursue our goals of the right to life. This would explain, the decision for example, by an ethics committee not to grant some British scientists who recently applied for permission to breed a human/cow hybrid, which they claim could offer opportunities to develop novel treatments for certain disorders. This example illustrates the point about not even science being perfect. As some would contend, the breach in the continuity of knowledge consequent upon the denial by the committee to grant the scientists permission to proceed with their projects is typical of the history of science itself, wherein the accumulated knowledge we now have one could say endowed 'philosophical value,' begs the question of the sanctity of scientific truth. Considering therefore, the sociological explanation that Kuhn adduced for the 'paradigmatic leaps' in 'revolutionary' versus 'normal' science even as the example above shows, the explanation applies to both, we confront directly the generic problem regarding the validity of scientific inquiry, regarding grounding the normative in the positive. This highlights the complexity resolving the semantics-from-syntax conundrum regarding 'meaning' not just pervasive in the cognitive paradigm, but hence worthy of our attention regarding the direction of the evolution of humankind. It is thus unclear whether the marketing push emergent wherein is not simply a question of commercials embedded in entertainment, there being actually blurring of the distinction between the two, with commercials, becoming entertainment orchestrated to remind the consumer of the brand that they surreptitiously advertise. In this context, should it surprise us that authorities in the U.S have given preliminary endorsement to a plan to grow rice modified genetically to produce human proteins, that we would soon see rice plants embedded with human genes involved in producing breast milk grown in Kansas[3]? As Ventria Bioscience, which made the proposal claimed the plants could become constituents of medications diarrhea and dehydration in infants, although there are concerns in certain quarters that the plants could mix with other drugs and enter the food chain, with potential adverse consequences for human health. That the proposal obtained preliminary support from the U.S Department of Agriculture does not necessarily mean that it would, the final approval, major regulatory obstacles in the way prior to food that contains human DNA being sold to consumers. Given the relatively common dearth of replication in research findings, particularly in the genetic association fields[4,5], it would be likely some would even question the 'science' of the rice. One survey of 600 positive associations between gene variants and common diseases noted consistent replication in just six of 166, reported associations[6]. Furthermore, the more scientific teams study a subject, the unlikelier the research findings from individual studies hold true[7]. Thus, we need to be vigorous in our efforts to pursue and to be as close to the truth as possible. Lest we lose focus of the fundamental truth we all must embrace, if humankind, as we know it, were not to find itself struggling some day for survival, in competition with for examples, the humanoids we created, whose fundamental objective might be different, or at least have nothing to do with the right to life. Our exploration therefore, predicated on at the very least the elements that have gotten us where we currently are, as the premise for our operations could not obviously be other than strategic, from our perspective. Thus, we could not afford to stifle competition in science and technology, for example, because we are averse to the emergence of hybrid forms, as they could be essential players in the realization of our objectives down the road. They might be able for instance to perform tasks, say walking through an inferno to shut off the controls of a leaking nuclear power plant, we are not best suited to do, or might prove not cost-effective or efficient for us to do and vice versa. Why then we would deny these alternate beings peaceful coexistence with us, not just, as they emerge but as they evolve into forms increasingly sophisticated, more than they were would be apposite to ask. Should our task not be to ensure that we are able to assure our right to life, rather than surrender this right perhaps intimidated by our co-inhabitants on the planet at the time, even if they did not coerce us into doing so, because of either larger numbers, or operations more intelligent and strategic, or based on social utility? It indeed, is also the case that our freedom or speech and expression, and indeed, of association, preclude us from doing otherwise, the outcomes of these freedoms, however, we must accept with humility, on the one hand, and visionary zeal on the other. These issues underscore the potential ramifications of the centrality of the healthcare consumer, or indeed, of the consumer, or the Copernican individual, going back full cycle, even if on a restricted scope, our planet. In other words, our exploration of this concept would lead us to the full realization of the need to inculcate it in persons from an early age, and to emphasize it at every phase of the life cycle, to ensure the measured approach to expression that would emerge on consensus as we apply those rights.

This constrained approach would be evident in not just our internal, but also our external affairs, as intellectual endowments become manifest across the globe. This would be more so, considering the potential ephemeral nature of our would-be co-inhabitants, despite the massive influence they might wield even so, in the hands of perhaps the most obscure of hands, whose control over them, they might eventually wrench, assuming the autonomy, defined by their own rules that we now enjoy. In other words, we have yet to fully exploit the benefits of the freedom we so cherish, those of the free market, that is evident is the way forward for all humankind, and of the institutions and infrastructures that underpin them, which every society would, as we become more cognizant of these benefits, embrace. Indeed, as we evolve, equipped with the knowledge of the potential of our freedoms to undermine us in the end, we 'embed' in our 'creations' a similar 'attitude' of self-respect and peaceful co-existence. Indeed, this would not be difficult not just for us to do, but for them to acquiesce, based on what we have understood is necessary for our survival in the end, which is to ensure that at every point in the evolution of our resources, we consider in full, what they portend for us, in the near-and long terms. The point then is that we could, with the elements of the free market operational par excellence, unleash the potential of those of our health systems to create the enabling milieu for the systems to contribute most effectively and efficiently to assuring the quality of the health of our peoples and the overall economic progress of our countries. We would under those circumstances not constrain ourselves by the considerations that do now, or any for that matter, in supporting efforts to ensure the manifestations of the interplay of the healthcare delivery/healthcare ICT dyadic, for example, in full. The technological progress that the ever-changing knowledge base of medical practice inspires in this instance, the bedrock of potential paradigmatic shifts in healthcare delivery, would ensure that each element of the dyadic feeds into each other in a catalytic symbiosis that would drive the motion of both forward. As noted earlier, our efforts regarding the widespread diffusion of these technologies would facilitate the full realization of the benefits of this interplay, at the individual and systemic levels, making it possible for us not to seem to have wasted the investments undoubted, substantial, we continue to make in our efforts to establish the technology infrastructure to complement such pervasiveness. In other words, as laudable as our efforts to build national health information networks are, these networks would not achieve their full potential, if for example, doctors and other healthcare professionals continue to have the current lackadaisical attitude towards these technologies. Yet, our prior efforts, based on the centrality of the healthcare consumer, would have made such undesirable results clear, preventing them in the first place. The preventive potential of our efforts as are those of our other initiatives are essentially work-in-progress. In short, we should not balk from them because we consider them unattainable, for example, because they are already here, and we cannot get everyone to purchase these technologies now. The fact is that our process cycle analyses, which incidentally these issues highlight, would reveal the appropriate initiatives for different contexts and persons that would be attainable, even if the emphasis on starting initiatives earlier remains. Thus, each life cycle would have issues that would require particular focus, under-age drinking for example, to the widespread nature of which the U.S acting Surgeon General Kenneth Moritsugu on March 6, 2007, alerted the country. Moritsugu described alcohol as the drug of choice for teens, according to the 2005 National Survey on Drug Use and Health estimates, 11 million underage drinkers in the country, almost 7.2 million, binge drinkers, that is who drank over five drinks on occasions. He called for action by all to tackle this menace, which is apt considering that whereas there has been a significant drop in tobacco and illicit drug use among teens, underage drinking remains highly prevalent. Indeed, we need to take prompt action, considering also its consequences being so dire, responsible for the deaths the acting Surgeon-General also noted of 5000 youths in the US alone every year, and according to one study, costs the country nearly $53 billion a year. This includes over $29 billion in alcohol-related violent crime costs, over $19 billion in traffic accidents, and over $1.5 billion in suicide attempts, both fatal and nonfatal[9]. The media glamorizing underage drinking for example would be another focus point, but this time, not directed at teenagers, which underscores the inter-connectedness of issues that we need to acknowledge and which should play a significant role in the initiatives we develop. We should therefore focus on our objectives to work within general and specific frameworks whose undercurrents coalesce to move our health systems forward, the general frameworks actually issues that would in effect apply to all health jurisdictions. In other words, those that are in the main mechanisms that those specific to particular jurisdictions would complement, which latter each jurisdiction would have to determine, again, via process cycle analyses of issues peculiar to them. Our discussion thus far thus stresses the multiplicity of domains that we need to explore in the health domain not failing to perform perhaps in the expectations of the healthcare consumer, even to surpass its mandates. In exploring these domains, would be our expectations to reveal their fundamental attributes, those pertinent to the realizations of these mandates, albeit many somewhat subterranean, to put them in perspective not just in relation to the status quo, but to revealed issues that would constitute new mandates in an ongoing quality improvement program. Our exploration therefore is an exercise in understanding the intricacies of the issues influencing healthcare delivery in a generic and specific sense, on the one hand, and of prescribing appropriate solutions to these issues on the other. Both elements of the exercise are important in themselves singly and together in achieving the dual healthcare delivery objectives mentioned earlier, which is crucial to any effort to ensure the health systems contributes substantially to the overall economic progress of society. We thus see our health system in broader terms than we currently do, making it likelier that we pursue the initiatives that would improve its operations. In other words, there is a congruence of motive and consequence, in teleological terms, which is not hedonic, although an element of which is constitutive of the right to life, but informed, as our prior efforts at rectifying information asymmetry mentioned earlier would ensure. Besides, in being just as cognizant of our obligations, our tendencies would be to conceptual healthcare delivery appropriately, formulating health policies cost-effectively, and efficiently to serve the interests of all, in so doing, account for the human and material, simultaneously, of the consequences of not so doing. It is the underlying assumption of the generic nature of our right to life that underpins this eclectic approach to healthcare delivery that health systems, worldwide would have to embrace in the new dispensation. In other words, a crucial aspect of the benefits of our exploration would be the understanding in full of the need for this approach and this would become more evident the more diffused, as we are able to inculcate the required knowledge and skills crucial to such understanding. This makes education the single most critical of the initiatives that we need to develop, the elements of which relevant to individuals, contextualized, more so realizing the disparities in the baseline among peoples from which we would start, these in personal and infrastructural terms. We would thus, need to establish programs simultaneously in both fronts, customized based on a variety of factors for particular health jurisdictions. Our efforts would also highlight the sometimes-subtle links between health and the economy and help clarify issues germane to service provision rooted in these links, for example, health financing, equity, and access to health services, among others. We would be able to see the significance of considerations of minority interests, and for the proper conceptualizations of the wealth of our country, in terms of not being just material, but also human or non-pecuniary. This way, the role of the delivery to all of qualitative and accessible health services would become even better appreciated by all echelons of society, the reasons for active and indeed, positive participation in the process that contribute to moving the health systems, hence the economy forward, more meaningful to all, guaranteeing such participation. It would therefore be most apposite, to create the enabling environment for such appreciation, and in effect be able to ensure the feeling of ownership of not just the health systems, but of the entire system around which our lives revolve. It is also clear therefore, that it would be the exact opposite to exclude anyone, minority, or others, from cultivating this feeling of ownership. Our exploration would therefore, enable us reformulate our approach to the integrity of society, fully aware of our commitments to its members, hence to formulate appropriate policies to deal with issues of immigration, in particular, as we realize the important input towards the economic progress of our countries that immigrants could contribute.

There is no doubt about the motion of forces along these lines, any denial of

the motorization of these forces in a different direction as possible as its potential ramifications are evident. It is in this context that we would for example, view the current debate in some quarters over mandating persons as Massachusetts in the U.S recently did, to purchase health insurance or face penalties. Besides the issues of enforceability, and the broadening by lobbyists potentially of the concept of insurance, which would swell the costs of the mandate with additional benefits consequently added, questions would arise regarding the potential to exclude rather than include certain persons, in particular the underprivileged. This is not to mention the potential increased health spending that government would face as such persons, who lacking bargaining power relative to the insurers, essentially lacking exit, would likely seek relief from government. Furthermore, would government likely not increase subsidies to meet such needs, with the potential for state funds to run out eventually, or cap insurance premiums, which would result in rationing health services, either of which could have adverse consequences for the healthcare consumer, the market and the economy? Thus, we confront the particular issues in our jurisdictions with comprehensive alacrity, knowing that we cannot delay finding the appropriate solutions to them, less they magnify, creating worse scenarios, which we would still have to address, anyway, and finding solutions to which would therefore, likely be more complicated, and costlier. In this particular instance, we would recognize that determining the goals to pursue is crucial, but so is finding the right answer. It would also remind us about the point regarding ownership we made earlier, as it would of the nature and extent of government participation in a free-market economy. Additionally, it would highlight the need to understanding fully, the significance of the interplay of the fundamentals some of which we have here discussed in nurturing this feeling of ownership on the one hand, and in revealing the need for starters and indeed, the effectiveness or otherwise of coercion in achieving goals that we all inherently seek, on the other. Is it possible for example that individuals would purchase health insurance without any government mandate to do so realizing the importance so doing to the overall economic progress of the country, for example, which having taken ownership of, assumes significance to them? This sense of ownership comes with a variety of institutional arrangements, and evident developments in the leadership hierarchy and in society in general that makes it difficult to achieve in some instances, and among certain individuals in society, currently. Yet, this only underscores the need to contextualize our efforts at rectifying information asymmetry, for example, delivering the right messages to individuals that would enable them, embrace this sense of ownership. This would make it unlikely to increase arousal that cognitive dissonance otherwise would[10], confronting the need to act accordingly, for example purchase health insurance, to protect the interest of what they own, protecting theirs. This does not necessarily confer these possibilities on the potential for rationality, as even the game theory, the key mathematics behind strategy, among others suggest that self-interest does not preclude short-term forfeitures for others' good, society providing the right milieu. Besides, considering self-interest in strict survivalist terms depletes it rationality, as it is absurd to argue that even cells come into being to die instantaneously, even those flawed from conception. This implies a certain universalization akin to Singer's meta-ethics, whose critique by Binmore, stressed the need for prior acceptance of all societies being equally important, placing significance to rationality of the sort we argue is not crucial for us to accept the primacy of the goals of improving our health systems for example, via improving our health, purchasing health insurance. In other words, our concept of contextualizing rectifying information asymmetry implies the disparities in the intellectual endowments of our peoples, in among other resources. It also implies that there would be those that would be unable to benefit from these efforts due to profound cognitive difficulties. Nonetheless, and as just as implicit in the idea is that of considering the interests of all, minorities included, and the clarity that not doing so would not be in anyone's best interest in the end. This underscores the need to ensure that our health services are accessible to all, and that they are qualitative and cost-effective, the support for the measures we take in this regard, having rectified information asymmetry, would enable their appreciation in full by those who could. Thus, our exploration would reveal in our jurisdictions the most appropriate ways to accomplish this critical goal, which generically would nonetheless involve efforts to achieve the dual healthcare delivery objectives mentioned earlier. Put differently, our efforts to achieve the DHDO would make it less problematic to achieve the delivery of qualitative healthcare cost-effectively and efficiently to all. It would be easier for us for example to accommodate initiatives that would ensure that all healthcare stakeholders gain, and not lose. We would in fact be able to advance the motion of our healthcare delivery faster, assuring its contribution to the overall progress of the national economy. Our efforts would enable the appreciation in full by the majority of such concepts as individual liberty, human dignity, and egalitarianism as the evident counter-intuitiveness of not so doing annuls any tendencies in that direction. It becomes clear that we could no longer advance society skewed in knowledge terms, and the options become ever starker, not doing something about it. Our exploration thus reveals the crossroads beyond which it is within our purview to advance, the realization of which would be the critical impetus for renewing our efforts to eschew the mundane and embrace the existential realities that seem to terrify us so intensely. We would attain the peace we so much cherish knowing that we have established the foundation for a better future for our loved ones and ourselves. Our finite form blends into the continuing evolution of humankind, and we as we embrace the sense of ownership of our country, feel a renewed vigor within that elevates our self-esteem. We start to see the beauty of humanity and its so-called 'dark-sides' become illusory, as if a bad dream we could wish away instantaneously. Yet, we acknowledge the transition that we have been through and that persists, consigning such dreams into the annals of history, reveling in our escape from the contraption of the crossroads. We would be cognizant of the tripartite possibilities we have, moving forward, backward or wobbling on the spot, indeed, collapsible into two, the potential acceleration or deceleration of the tendency to wobble on the spot, one of two options of dissipating eventually or changing position. We would then realize that in effect, we could choose to move forward or backward, in the direction of life or be moribund. That we would choose the latter is possible but implausible given as we noted earlier that even flawed organisms fight expiration. Why then should we delay in initiating action on assuring the motion in the appropriate direction of our affairs and systems? The cacophony that seemingly simply diffuses in the ethereal now would become increasingly coherent and would not just raise such questions even more but also proffer solutions to them, as we become increasingly suave in our understanding of the relevant issues that our explorations engender. Indeed, it might just be that we are about to shift gear, and change position given that we could not be stuck at the crossroads, in which direction we head, though, we would have to decide.

References:

1. Available at:
http://www.nytimes.com/2007/03/02/washington/02poll.html?_r=2&adxnnl=1&or
ef=slogin&ref=todayspaper&adxnnlx=1172854800-
P38Y6lVXPm2ZPHHiIj5W2g&pagewanted=print Accessed on March 04, 2007

2. Paul S (1992). Accountability in public services: exit, voice, and control. World Development 20(7): 1047-60

3. Available at: http://news.bbc.co.uk/2/hi/americas/6422297.stm Accessed on March 6, 2007

4. Cardon LR, Bell JI (2001) Association study designs for complex diseases. Nat Rev Genet 2: 91–99.

5. Redden DT, Allison DB (2003) Nonreplication in genetic association studies of obesity and diabetes research. J Nutr 133: 3323–3326.

6. Hirschhorn JN, Lohmueller K, Byrne E, Hirschhorn K (2002) A comprehensive review of genetic association studies. Genet Med 4: 45–61.

7. Ioannidis JPA (2005) Why most published research findings are false. PLoS Med 2: 124–doi:10.1371/journal.pmed.0020124 doi:10.1371/journal.pmed.0020124.

8. Available at:

http://www.msnbc.msn.com/id/17491440/wid/11915773?GT1=9145 Accessed on
March 7, 2007

9. Levy, D.T., Miller, T. R., Spicer, R., & Stewart, K. *Underage Drinking:
Intermediate Consequences and their Costs*, Pacific Institute for Research and
Evaluation working paper, June 1999.

10. Festinger, L., and Carlsmith, J. M. (1959). "Cognitive consequences of forced
compliance". *Journal of Abnormal and Social Psychology*, 58, 203-211.
Available at: http://psychclassics.yorku.ca/Festinger/index.htm
Accessed on March 7, 2007.

11. Singer, P. *The Expanding Circle: Ethics and Sociobiology*, New York: Farrar,
Straus and Giroux, 1981, ISBN 0-374-23496-5.

12. Binmore, K. *Natural Justice*, Oxford: Oxford University Press, 2005. ISBN 0-19-
517811-4.

Conclusion

Our task as evident in our exploration is an urgent attention to our vision of

delivering accessible and qualitative health services to all. It is also clear that the logistics of achieving this goal would vary according to health jurisdictions, as it is that a generic framework within which these jurisdictions could operate is critical to appreciate and accept. Our exploration also reveals our potential to change our current practices to achieve our desired healthcare delivery goals. It reveals the underlying forces that drive our interests in protecting our right to life, forces whose interplay in forging our vision of not just healthcare delivery, but also its interplay with other forces in determining our ability to move our economy forward is critical to appreciate, fully.

In our ever-competitive world, with globalization ensuring the mobility of

labor, technological progress, realigning the nature and ubiquity of employment, and the knowledge and skills inherent in human capital veritable sources of wealth creation in contemporary economies, the fact that we need to situate this right in the context of change, is evident. That it is urgent that we need to address the cross-domain issues on which healthcare delivery would increasingly hinge, for example the crucial role of increasing human capital, on the one hand, and of improving its quality, including in the health domain, on the other is just as clear. We could no longer for example dismiss the need to be cognizant of the healthcare requirements of the immigrants we allow into our countries to buoy our workforce. Nor could we rest assured that by giving them enough wages, we would have played our part in the reciprocal enterprise of labor employment, knowing that by being in our countries, means we could not afford to ignore the needs of their wives and children as well, so doing with potential adverse consequences for ours.

Our exploration would thus, have broadened our perspective of the deeper

linings of healthcare delivery, and the need to pay increasing attention to them. It would also have alerted us to the promise of healthcare delivery in our economic progress at the individual and national levels that we could not even contemplate frittering. Perhaps most cogently, we would have realized the immense benefits accruable from the exercise itself that is our exploration, given, what some might consider the discouraging stealth it might initially present. This would ensure that we do not dither in applying similar principles to other aspects of our affairs, to elucidate underpinnings that could motivate us in visualizing the mundane less pithily. This is because the application of rigor oftentimes unpleasant, albeit not for all, could be the antidote to the persistence of even more disagreeable developments in our health systems.

In recognizing as we have in our discussions of the chances of no health system

being perfect, for example, we would be keen to make ours as close to perfection as we possibly could. Yet, we would acknowledge the need for ongoing process cycle analyses that would via continuous decomposition and exposition, highlight the salient issues that particular health jurisdictions need to tackle, and indeed, the solutions to them. That these analyses would assume the malleability of the system, and the need to stay ahead of the disruptions that change would visit on it, which need urgent attention to ensure the system's continuing ability to deliver qualitative health services efficiently and cost-effectively, would be sufficient for us to perpetuate them. Thus, our exploration would have inculcated in us the need for thoroughness and rigor that the issues at hand demand for effective solutions to emerge and move them forward. There is no doubt that these issues might seem impossible to achieve given the present dispensation, in other words, with the current widespread information asymmetry worldwide, but we would be confident in our abilities so to do given the appreciation of the issues the exploration affords. Thus, and in a more generic sense, the presence of, and the nature and extent of the obstacles in the way of achieving our objectives in our particular jurisdictions would not be sufficient, as would nothing really, to faze us.

This is because, and as our exploration has revealed, we derive an inner strength in the full realization of the very reasons for which we live, and the critical nature of our efforts in supporting them that would be sufficient in scaling whatever obstacles seem to threaten to deny us that chance. It would be apposite for us therefore to promote such explorations as could so equip us to initiate such significant changes in our health systems that would be in keeping with our stated objectives of delivering qualitative health services to all cost-effectively and efficiently. In other words, crucial to realizing the promise of our exploration is ensuring that others engage in similar exercises, which would be a most efficient way to move closer to achieving our goals, and faster too. As we have observed thus far, it is time we started to see healthcare delivery in its true ramifications, as an important aspect of ensuring our right to life, on the one hand, and of that of our economy to thrive, if not in fact, survive, on the other. This appreciation of the importance of health and of healthcare delivery is an essential aspect of our efforts to move the motion of our affairs as humans forward, a motion, which we have control over, which itself assures us of the freedom we so much desire being not impossible to achieve, as some contend, but actually inherent in us all.

Healthcare would no doubt play an increasingly significant role in our affairs

in the years ahead. This, among other reasons, means that we need to understand fully the forces at play in shaping it. Some of these forces would be dynamic, others static, but they would all, singly and in combination require our attention in appreciating how we could maneuver them to contribute positively to the achievement of our dual healthcare delivery objectives (DHDO). We would no longer have any excuse to allow our health systems to drift aimlessly as they currently do as though we could not steer them in the direction that we wish. As our exploration has shown, we have control over these forces, and should be able to make them work for us, but we must understand them. It would be much easier for us to tame them if we did. Indeed, we would have no choice but so to do, as we increasingly also realize that it is unsustainable for us to continue, for example, to spend increasing amounts on health, while not benefiting from these huge investments to the extent that we should. In other words, the need for such explorations as we have thus far advocated would become increasingly clear, as we understand and are able to better relate the fundamentals of the workings of our health systems vis-à-vis those of our very existence to our present and future realities, even more.

As is clear from our discussion in the e-book that ensuring that we improve

our health systems is the business of us all, it behooves us therefore, to embark on efforts in our different capacities that we could make to contribute to the realization of this goal. In short, we would have achieved an important objective of this e-book, and the time we have expended in reading it worthwhile if we did. There is no doubt that we could make a difference to health services delivery in our particular jurisdiction, exercising the prerogative what we have imbibed in our discussions here confers. That we acknowledge the potential of our contribution towards improving the health system as a whole is testimony to such an exercise in the making, which actualizing in whatever way we could essentially completes the cycle. This is not to say that our efforts should a one-off matter. In fact, as we have also seen in our discussions here, it is a continuous quality assurance process, the contribution to which by all of us is the most apposite in achieving.

Copyright Bankix Systems Ltd March 8, 2007

9 781703 732238